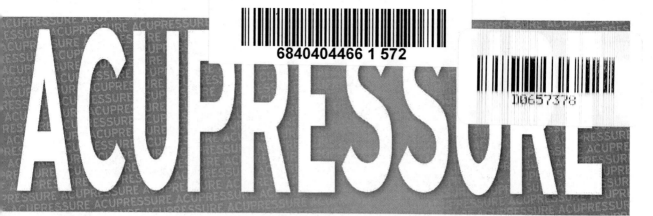

ACUPRESSURE

The Essential Guide

Denis Jevon

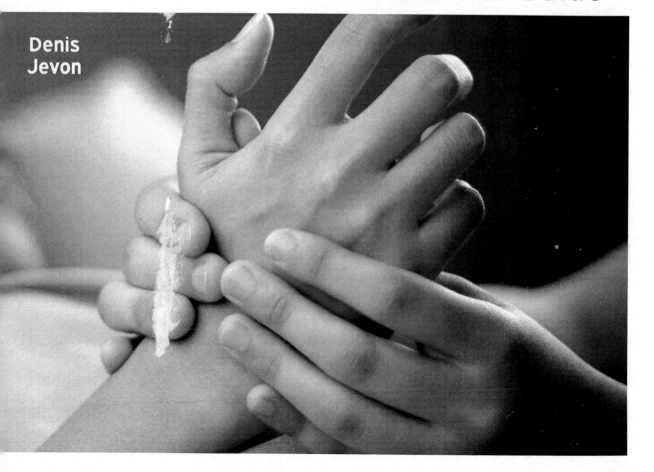

Acupressure: The Essential Guide is also available in accessible formats for people with any degree of visual impairment. The large print edition and e-book (with accessibility features enabled) are available from Need2Know. Please let us know if there are any special features you require and we will do our best to accommodate your needs.

First published in Great Britain in 2012 by
Need2Know
Remus House
Coltsfoot Drive
Peterborough
PE2 9BF
Telephone 01733 898103
Fax 01733 313524
www.need2knowbooks.co.uk

Contents

Introduction

Acupressure is a subtle healing art based on principles that are thousands of years old.

In the East, acupressure is part of a system of healing that has been studied and documented throughout the ages. In many places it is still relied upon as a major part of health care right through to the present day.

Ki, the life-giving energy

The human body is so much more than a mass of bones, tissues, blood and organs. It is more than the thoughts, feelings and nerve impulses that are recognised by Western science and medicine. In the East it has long been understood that a subtle energy, 'ki' in Japanese, 'qi' (pronounced 'chee') in Chinese, exists within all living things. Ki is the life-force energy which animates all aspects of nature. Although ki infuses the whole body, it tends to flow through channels called meridians. The points used in acupressure and acupuncture exist mostly on these meridians.

When ki is in harmony the organism is healthy. When it is out of balance mental, physical, emotional or spiritual ill health can occur. Pressure on certain points helps to restore the harmonious flow of ki through the meridians. This is the fundamental principle behind acupressure and allied healing arts.

This book aims to give an insight into the background and practice of acupressure throughout its long history. In order to help explain the philosophy behind Oriental medicine the reader is introduced to the concepts of yin and yang, the Five Elements and Oriental Diagnosis. It is not necessary to have a deep knowledge of these things to be able to use acupressure. However, for those who are interested, it gives some insight into aspects of how this ancient system works.

'The human body is so much more than a mass of bones, tissues, blood and organs.'

The various therapies based on acupressure will be introduced and explained with examples of ways in which they can help common health problems. There is a strong emphasis on the complementary nature of acupressure treatments and how they can work alongside modern Western medicine and other complementary therapies.

Self-help

The second part of the book is a self-help resource to enable the reader to use simple acupressure techniques to help themselves, their family and friends. This does not in any way attempt to be a replacement for conventional medical treatment. Medical advice should always be sought. There are comprehensive descriptions of how to find and use acupressure points, along with diagrams and illustrations.

There are over 350 documented acupressure points in the human body and only a selection are used in this book. Easily located ones are suggested and no equipment is required to locate or stimulate the points. The acupressure techniques and points described are selected from those traditionally used for self-help. These are safe and effective and can often help with problems such as headaches, nausea, period pain, muscle cramps, aches and pains, and much more.

I hope that this book will inspire an interest that will continue, as mine has, for a lifetime. Perhaps some readers will even go on to study further or to train as a therapist. Suggestions are made for further study or how to find a practitioner. Most of all I hope that this essential guide to acupressure will fascinate, inform and help you, the reader.

Disclaimer

This book is for general information about acupressure. Anyone experiencing ongoing health problems should first see their health professional. It is important to reach a diagnosis, then establish the most appropriate form of treatment.

The pressure points and techniques described in *Acupressure: The Essential Guide* are contemporary interpretations of traditional methods that have been in use in the Orient for thousands of years. Nothing in this book is intended to constitute a prescription or to supersede or replace any Western first aid or medical treatment.

Part 1

Chapter One

Acupressure: An Overview

What is acupressure?

Acupressure is often referred to as 'acupuncture without needles'. Like acupuncture, acupressure works on the principle that the universe is permeated by a subtle energy called 'ki'. In humans and animals, ki fills the whole being and mostly travels through channels referred to as meridians. Meridians are divided into surface meridans and deep meridans (internal). Acupressure points are located on the surface meridians. These points are the same ones that needles are inserted into in acupuncture.

While ki is flowing correctly through all the meridians then a healthy state is maintained. When the flow of ki is blocked or weakened then a state of ill health can exist. Applying pressure to the correct points restores the flow of ki in the meridians, thereby encouraging good health or enhanced energy.

'While ki is flowing correctly through all the meridians then a healthy state is maintained. When the flow of ki is blocked or weakened then a state of ill health can exist.'

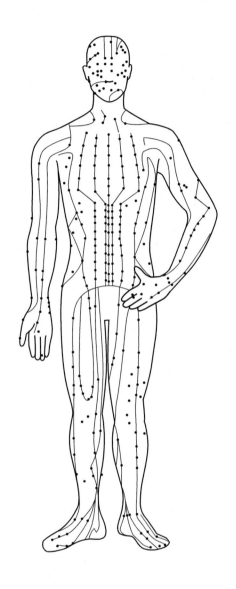

How did acupressure start?

One of the most natural responses to pain or discomfort is touch. If you have a headache, stomach ache or if you hit your thumb with a hammer, the first reaction is to hold or rub the affected part. Equally, if a child has a pain the parent will instinctively place a comforting hand on them. This instinctive impulse of the soothing touch may be where massage and acupressure had their origins. It is not too hard to imagine that pressure points were discovered over a long period of time more or less by accident. As an example, someone may have had a problem with a muscle spasm or cramp and accidently stimulated a pressure point that gave them instant relief.

Gifted therapists can often sense the energy difference of a pressure point and thereby its location. It is likely that sensitive practitioners in times gone by located new pressure points in this way. During treatments clients sometimes give feedback that when a point is pressed they can feel a sensation along the pathway of the meridian. This is another way in which meridians may have been mapped. It is not hard to imagine that the range of symptoms that can be relieved by pressing a particular pressure point were discovered through curiosity, experimentation and experience. All this feedback must have contributed to the accumulation of knowledge in the past.

There are old Chinese stories that acupuncture points were sometimes discovered when a soldier was wounded in a particular place by an arrow or sword. Later, the person would find that some chronic symptom had disappeared. That symptom would then be associated with the point. Knowledge of the location and uses of pressure points were undoubtedly passed down and added to over many generations as were the different techniques used to stimulate pressure points. All this has built into the body of knowledge that exists today.

Ki – the life force

The universal life force is called 'ki' (pronounced 'kee') in Japanese and 'qi' (pronounced 'chee') in Chinese. Eastern philosophy divides ki into yin and yang. Yin is the expansive outward and upward moving energy and yang is the contracting, inward and downward moving energy. Yin and yang are relative terms and things are described as more yin or more yang. Sometimes interpretations of yin and yang vary slightly. This book is written from the perspective of a more Japanese influence and training. Here are some examples:

Category	More Yin	More Yang
Movement	More inactive, slower	More active, faster
Direction	Upward and outward	Downward and inward
Weight	Lighter	Heavier
Size	Larger	Smaller
Texture	Softer	Harder
Climate	Hotter	Colder
Food type	Vegetable	Meat
Type of work	More mental	More physical
Gender	Female	Male
Emotion	More gentle	More forceful
Mental attitude	More forward-looking	More backward-looking

'To the Oriental way of thinking all things are made up of a combination of five elements: Water, Metal, Earth, Wood and Fire.'

Furthermore, to the oriental way of thinking all things are made up of a combination of five elements: Water, Wood, Fire, Earth and Metal. Wood is sometimes referred to as Tree.

In acupressure there are fourteen main meridians. These are divided into yin and yang and each meridian belongs to one of the five elements. Each meridian controls and is associated with an organ or body system. These are recognisable within the Western view of the human body with a couple of exceptions. The table that follows shows these meridians.

Meridian Name	Yin/Yang	Element	Organ/system
Central Vessel	Yin	All or none	Brain
Governing Vessel	Yang	All or none	Central nervous system
Stomach	Yang	Earth	Stomach
Spleen/Pancreas	Yin	Earth	Spleen or pancreas
Heart	Yin	Fire	Cardiovascular system
Small Intestine	Yang	Fire	Small intestine
Bladder	Yang	Water	Urinary tract and bladder
Kidney	Yin	Water	Kidneys
Heart Protector	Yin	Fire	Pericardium and circulation
Triple Heater	Yang	Fire	Thyroid and metabolism
Gall Bladder	Yang	Wood	Gall bladder
Liver	Yin	Wood	Liver
Lung	Yin	Metal	Lung
Large Intestine	Yang	Metal	Large intestine

The Central Vessel (or Conception Vessel) and the Governing Vessel are not considered part of the Five Element system and are not associated with an element. They are the connection between the universal ki energy and the individual's meridian system. They are the pathways through which the ki of the universe feeds into the human being. The kidneys are similarly considered as an interface between the universal and human life force.

The two meridians that have no obvious equivalent in Western medicine are the Heart Protector and the Triple Warmer. The Heart Protector controls circulation of blood and ki. It can affect things like blood pressure and heart rate as well as the general level of energy or vitality. The Triple Warmer regulates body temperature and is associated with metabolism and some of the endocrine gland functions.

The Five Elements

In the ancient world attempts were made to make sense of what everything was made from, and to describe the forces of nature. In the West there were four basic elements, Earth, Air, Fire and Water. In the East the elements were described as Earth, Wood or Tree, Fire, Metal and Water. As well as being the constituents of everything, the Five Elements are linked by a cycle of transformation. Water feeds Tree, making it grow. Wood burns creating Fire. Fire leaves behind ash or Earth. Earth is compressed to form Metal. Water condenses on Metal.

The following table shows some of the qualities associated with each of the Five Elements. The preceding table and this one can be used together to help decide which pressure points to use for a particular problem. For example, there are many different points which can be used to relieve a headache. If you have headaches when you have been out in windy conditions or in a draught, you might choose a pressure point which is governed by the element Wood, in other words on the gall bladder or liver meridian. This is because Wood is associated with windy conditions. Whereas if the headaches are associated with a lot of nasal mucus and sinus pain then Metal may be the element that is out of balance. If the bowels were out of sorts as well (constipation, diarrhoea or intestinal gas) then you might choose points on the large intestine meridian.

Element	Earth	Wood	Fire	Metal	Water
Organ	Spleen, pancreas	Liver, gall bladder	Heart, small intestine	Lungs, large intestine	Kidneys, bladder
Opening	Mouth	Eyes	Ears	Nose	Anus, urinary
Parts of body	Flesh, lips	Muscles, nails	Pulse, complexion	Skin, body hair	Bones, hair on head
Fluid	Lymph	Tears	Sweat	Mucus	Saliva
Odour	Sweet	Rancid	Burnt	Fleshy	Putrid
Taste	Sweet	Acid	Bitter	Piquant	Salty
Sense	Taste	Sight	Speech	Smell	Hearing
Emotions	Worry	Anger	Joy	Grief	Fear
Colour	Yellow	Blue	Red	White	Black
Sound	Singing	Crying	Laughing	Sobbing	Groaning
Climate	Damp	Wind	Heat	Dryness	Cold

Need2Know

Acupressure therapies

Throughout the centuries many different therapies have developed that use acupressure. Some use only thumb or fingertip pressure directly on the pressure points. Whereas other therapies focus less directly on the pressure points and use massage for a more diffused stimulation of the meridians. Some therapies use the elbow, palm, heel of the hand, forearm, knuckles or foot to stimulate the meridians or pressure points. Others use a specially shaped stone or wooden tool to work on meridians and points.

Acupressure therapies available today include:

* Anma.

* Shiatsu.

* Jin Shin Jyutsu.

* Tuina.

* Applied Kinesiology.

* TFT.

* EFT.

* Seated Acupressure Massage.

There are many other types of therapy which are based on or include acupressure techniques. However, those mentioned show quite well the variety of approaches to acupressure and the diverse ways in which it has developed.

* Anma – Anma is one of the oldest forms of acupressure treatment. It originated in Central and Northern parts of China thousands of years ago where it was known as Anmo. It uses a variety of pressing, squeezing, stretching and other techniques applied with the hands, fingers, forearms, knuckles and elbows. Anma is the earliest type of massage/acupressure to be actually recorded, around 2,500 years ago. It is thought to have started between 5,000 and 10,000 years ago.

* Shiatsu – Shiatsu is related to and grew out of Anma in the early twentieth century and has become a separate therapy with the addition of many

'Throughout the centuries many different therapies have developed that use acupressure.'

techniques. Variants such as Healing Shiatsu have become available over recent years with the rise in popularity of complementary medicine in the West.

- Jin Shin Jyutsu – Jin Shin Jyutsu only uses 26 pressure points, whereas there are over 300 used in Anma and Shiatsu. The practitioner uses both hands to hold combinations of pressure points to bring about a harmonious state of being.

- Tuina – Tuina has a history of at least 1,700 years. It works along the path of the meridians and rather than applying finger pressure to specific points, tuina uses friction and kneading. In this way it is similar to Western styles of massage. It is also said to resemble chiropractic and osteopathy. Tuina is commonly used to relieve muscle and joint pain. It works by redistributing ki from and to areas where there is an excess or a deficiency of this energy.

- Applied Kinesiology – Applied Kinesiology came about in the 1960s in America. It is a method of assessing the status of the meridians using muscle testing. Pressure points and other methods are then used to restore balance to the energy systems. Many forms of therapy have developed over the years based on this principle and continue to do so.

- TFT (Thought Field Therapy) – TFT was developed by Dr. Roger Callaghan in 1979 and it is a continuing process. TFT is a sequential tapping procedure. Pressure points are tapped in a particular sequence depending on the diagnosed problem. TFT uses different algorhythms or sequences of points for specific problems. It claims a high success rate in many situations including post-traumatic stress disorder (PTSD) and many other psycho-emotional problems.

- EFT (Emotional Freedom Technique) – EFT is a relative newcomer and was started in the early 1990s by Gary Craig. It was derived from TFT. EFT uses a limited number of acupressure points which are treated with rhythmic tapping. While tapping the points phrases are repeated in order to balance the ki of the client in relation to a particular emotional state. This 'resets' the meridians to a more harmonious state and symptoms are alleviated. EFT is used for a wide range of problems including phobia, PTSD, anger management, physical pain and even restrictions in physical movement. It is one of a range of new therapies known as Meridian Energy Techniques.

- Seated Acupressure Massage – Seated Acupressure is a fairly new application of acupressure techniques derived from Anma. Usually a kata, a series of moves, is used to apply treatment to meridians and pressure points. The areas treated are mostly the back, shoulders, arms and head. The client is seated in a specially designed and very comfortable massage chair for the treatment, hence the name. Seated Acupressure treatments can be invaluable in situations where a client cannot lie down due to severe back or neck problems. Because the client does not have to remove clothing and the chair is very portable, this treatment can be performed in all sorts of situations, for instance in the office, on a cruise liner, in an airport lounge and so on.

More detail on some of these therapies is given in chapter 3.

Uses of acupressure

Acupressure is very versatile and in its many forms it can be applied to any number of different situations. There are times when an acupressure treatment can be given as first aid (not replacing Western style first aid, but as an adjunct) to relieve acute symptoms or problems. Equally, there are clients who can be helped through long-term or chronic problems through regular treatments. The different forms of acupressure lend themselves to different styles of application, however all styles would undoubtedly claim a wide range of uses.

'Acupressure is very versatile and in its many forms it can be applied to any number of different situations.'

A traditional tale

There is a story of a young Japanese woman who did not get on with her mother-in-law and wished her dead. She went to a wise Shiatsu practitioner who told her that if she was serious she should give her mother-in-law a daily Shiatsu treatment accompanied by a herb tea. The young woman did this for six months and in the process got to know her mother-in-law and no longer wished her dead. In fact she grew to understand her. She returned to the master and asked him how she could reverse the process. He said that there was no need. The Shiatsu had helped to form a bond between them and the herb tea was completely harmless.

This is a lovely example of the way in which interaction through a physical therapy can form a healing bond over a period of time. The following case illustrates well how acupressure can sometimes give almost instant relief from a long-standing problem.

Case study

A physically active male in his early fifties presented with a great deal of pain in his back and severely limited movement. He related that he had suffered this problem for fifteen years since a rugby injury. After taking a brief case history he was given a twenty-minute Seated Acupressure treatment to the back, arms, neck and shoulders. At the end of the treatment he had complete relief from the symptoms and full movement was restored. Years later there has been no recurrence of the problem.

'Mental, physical, emotional and spiritual problems can all be helped by the skilled application of acupressure.'

These two examples illustrate the different ends of the spectrum in terms of the ways in which various forms of acupressure can work. There are many different applications of these healing arts that fall all along that spectrum. Mental, physical, emotional and spiritual problems can all be helped by the skilled application of acupressure. Equally, very basic self-help acupressure can prove to be invaluable in minor, acute or emergency situations.

Self-help or professional consultation?

There are many situations where it is advisable to seek the help of a practitioner, sometimes, however, self-help is more appropriate. If you have a problem which has a known cause – for instance stage fright or muscle cramps through over-exercise – then self-help acupressure or EFT may be appropriate. Conversely, in chronic illness or where there is a complex underlying emotional situation it may be wise to consult a professional. Factors that need considering are:

- Should you see, or have you seen a doctor?
- Is this a long-term problem?
- Is this a 'one-off' situation?
- Do you know why you are suffering?

- Are you out of your depth?

- Is your problem physical, emotional, mental or spiritual?

- Is help readily available?

- Can you get to a doctor or hospital in reasonable time?

- Can you phone emergency services?

The list is potentially endless. In the end common sense must come into play. However it cannot be emphasised enough, if in doubt see a doctor or visit A&E. It is no good using acupressure, especially if you are a layperson, when you are having a heart attack or have a broken hip.

Some of the problems treatable with acupressure

- Insect bites and stings (unless you have an allergic reaction).

- Headaches.

- Colds and flu.

- Period pain.

- Poor circulation, chilblains.

- Toothache (when you can't get to a dentist).

- Phobias and fears.

- Anxiety.

- Allergies.

- Indigestion.

- Muscle aches and spasms.

- Exhaustion.

- Feeling cold.

- Sinus and nasal congestion.

- Constipation.
- Lack of energy.
- Flatulence.
- Hangover.
- Feeling overly hot.
- Indigestion.
- Poor memory.
- Nausea.
- Restlessness.
- Stopping smoking.
- Stiff neck.
- Yawning.

If symptoms persist consult your health-care practitioner.

This is not a complete list and there are many other problems that acupressure may be able to help with. If this means you take fewer chemical drugs into your body then so much the better. Obviously there are many times when the use of chemicals, or other medicines, are very helpful and essential. If, however, they can be avoided it puts less strain on the system.

If you fall whilst walking or climbing alone on a remote hillside and are in great pain, for instance, and you could have a long wait for help, then acupressure to relieve pain or to warm your body would be invaluable. Equally, if you are at the theatre or at an opera and you have a hiccupping attack, then knowing a way to stop it may save you a lot of embarrassment!

Summing Up

▪ Acupressure has been used extensively for many thousands of years. There are many forms of acupressure, some ancient and others more modern. All are based along similar lines.

▪ Acupressure is based on the principle that a subtle energy 'ki' (Japanese) or 'qi' (Chinese) flows through channels in the body called meridians. On these meridians are pressure points. By applying stimulation to these points and meridians, the practitioner seeks to bring about positive changes in the health of the client. This restores or balances the flow of ki.

▪ Ki is the universal and individual life force that is divided into yin and yang and the Five Elements.

▪ By learning some basic techniques and the location of some points, self-help using acupressure is possible. Acupressure is not a replacement for Western medicine but can work effectively alongside it or when it is unavailable.

Chapter Two

Oriental Diagnosis

An oriental view of the cosmos

One of the fundamental differences between the typical European/American (i.e. 'Western') view of the cosmos and the 'Eastern' is the concept of 'ki' or 'chi'. Ki is the universal energy that flows through and animates all things from galaxies to microscopic organisms.

In recent years, scientific research is showing that when we look at matter at very high magnification, so-called solid matter is composed of tiny particles with large expanses of empty space in-between. Furthermore, if those particles are examined more closely it turns out that they are also mostly made up of empty space scattered with even smaller particles. What holds all these particles in place within these expanses of empty space? Energy. In fact the particles themselves appear to be made of energy and some of them even seem to flicker in and out of existence, changing into energy and then back to matter! So those Oriental scholars of long ago seem to have got it right. All things are infused with and are in fact made from energy, or ki as they called it.

Yin, yang and transformation

One of the basic laws of physics, attributed to Sir Isaac Newton, is that 'energy cannot be created or destroyed, it can only be transferred from one form to another'. Likewise, in the Oriental scheme of things energy is constantly changing form. Ki is divided into 'yin' and 'yang' and all things are composed of varying proportions of yin and yang. Nothing in the universe is static and everything is in a state of flux, constantly changing form. This is most obvious in the natural world where things come into being, grow, change and eventually decay, returning back to where they came from.

'One of the basic laws of physics, attributed to Sir Isaac Newton, is that "energy cannot be created or destroyed, it can only be transferred from one form to another".'

Yin and yang are opposite yet complementary. One cannot exist without the other. Nothing is totally yang or yin. All things are made up of varying proportions of these two. All things are further divided into the Five Elements which are in a state of transformation from one to another. As we saw in chapter 1 the different organs and systems of the human body are associated with different elements and meridians, and are considered to be more yin or more yang in nature. In diagnosis all these factors are taken into account along with things like the time of day when symptoms occur, the season, whether the person is in a hot or cold situation, or if they have been affected by wind, rain or other extremes. Oriental Diagnosis, an art and specialism in itself, can be very complex and subtle and is a lifetime's study. There are, however, some obvious diagnostic signs which would help someone decide which pressure points would help them.

Face diagnosis

One of the widely held beliefs in oriental medicine is that individual parts of the body can represent the whole and that the whole body can be treated through one small part. A good example of this is face diagnosis where the shape of the face and the size, shape and colouration of various features can give insight into the state of the organs and systems of the body. The diagram that follows is a map of the main areas of the face and the organs they represent according to tradition.

'One of the widely held beliefs in oriental medicine is that individual parts of the body can represent the whole and that the whole body can be treated through one small part.'

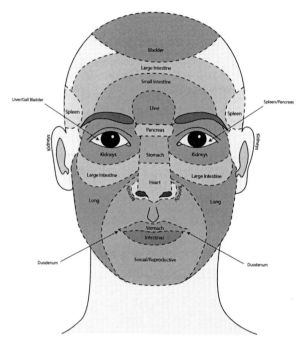

White of left eye = Spleen/Pancreas

White of right eye = Liver/Gall bladder

Corbers of mouth = Duodenum

Other indicators

- Large, well formed ear lobes (as shown on many statues of Buddha) are a sign of a good constitution.

- A well-defined, deep and strong philtrum (the vertical groove between the nose and upper lip) is a sign of strong sexual energy.

- The length and bushiness of the eyebrows is a sign of longevity and vigour.

Reading the face

Faces come in all shapes, sizes and proportions. So it is necessary to make adjustments and allowances for these differences. The face map shown can only be a guide to the areas representing different organs on any particular face.

The face, like any other part of the body, can give us clues to the constitution and the condition of the person.

- Constitution is the underlying nature of the person, governed by inherited factors, the way the body was formed in the womb and during early life.

- Condition is the effect of diet, lifestyle, stresses and strains of life, etc.

The shape of the face as a whole and the relative shapes and proportions of the different areas show constitutional factors. Things like skin colour and texture, spots and blemishes, hairs and warts are conditional factors.

Both can be helpful indicators in different ways.

- Constitutional signs on the face can give you insight into your strengths and weaknesses, enabling you to know which systems and organs you will need to take extra care of.

- Conditional signs can give you early warning that a problem may be brewing in a particular area.

For instance, someone with relatively small ears and/or eyes may have constitutional weakness of the kidneys. They would be advised to make sure that they avoid overstressing the kidneys with coffee, tea and alcohol, and to guard against becoming dehydrated. Whereas a person who starts to regularly get puffy, watery bags under the eyes or dark rings around and under the eyes is undergoing a lot of stress to the kidneys. This shows conditional change rather than constitutional factors. If this coincides with strong, dark urine they would be well advised to see a doctor to check kidney function.

The following sections give insight into the individual areas of the face.

'The face, like any other part of the body, can give us clues to the constitution and the condition of the person.'

The forehead

The forehead can suffer with dry areas, spots, rashes and other irritations. Depending on where these arise they can show problems with the organs or systems connected with that area. For instance:

- If the area associated with the spleen (just above the temples) is spotty or itchy this can show some overload in the lymphatic system due to infection or toxicity.

- If spots or redness regularly appear in the central forehead it means that the small intestine is probably being overloaded with animal fats in the diet or the gall bladder is not working efficiently enough to help digest those fatty foods.

The ears

Ears in general represent the kidneys. The size of the ears as a whole reflects the size and efficiency of the kidneys.

- Small ears may mean smaller and less efficient kidneys which need to be looked after.

- Hot or red ears can be the sign of a kidney infection.

- Tinnitus, itchy ears and hair growth in the ear canals are often associated with imbalances of the kidneys, possible toxicity or inappropriate diet.

The eyes

Eyes and the area around them also represent the kidneys and to some degree the adrenal glands. The adrenals sit on top of the kidneys and interact with them. The adrenal glands have many important functions. They produce the hormones adrenalin associated with the 'fight or flight' reaction, and cortisol which is released in response to stress.

- Dark colouration around the eyes, bloodshot eyes and puffy eyelids or bags under the eyes all show problems with the kidneys. The problem could be insufficient intake of water, excess of salt or alcohol, or kidney disease or damage. If the symptoms continue for a long time a more serious kidney problem may be developing.

- Dark colouration around the eyes, oversensitivity to bright light can also show the adrenal glands are overworked.

- If the whites of the eyes have a yellow discolouration this reflects a liver problem and if the colouration is very obvious or continues medical help must be sought.

- The white of the left eye is associated with the spleen and the right one with the liver and gall bladder.

- Some people have small creamy white marks on the white of the eye that are slightly raised from the surface of the eye, these are known as 'cheese spots'. These are said to show an excessive intake of dairy products over a long period, or that the person does not process dairy foods very well. It is a good idea to avoid eating large amounts of dairy produce (especially cow's milk and cheese) in this case.

'Eyes and the area around them represent the kidneys and to some degree the adrenal glands.'

Sanpaku

In Japanese 'Sanpaku' literally means 'three whites'. It refers to the areas of white of the eyes that are normally visible. In most people the white areas at the sides of the iris are usually visible. In some people the white area above the iris or below it is also visible most of the time. These conditions are known as 'Yin Sanpaku' and 'Yang Sanpaku'.

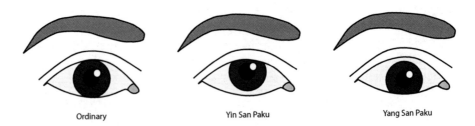

Ordinary   Yin San Paku   Yang San Paku

Yin Sanpaku denotes a more yin constitution. Particularly, it can mean a less vigorous and active approach to life and a tendency towards weakness physically or mentally. Yin Sanpaku can be caused by excess of yin foods, alcohol or drugs. These are conditional factors. Some people are just born with an extremely yin constitution and may naturally be yin Sanpaku.

Yang Sanpaku denotes a more yang constitution. People with this diagnostic sign are strong physically and are very determined or tough. Mentally they can be quite rigid. Some authorities say that yang Sanpaku people are prone to violence or aggression. Yang Sanpaku can be brought about by an excessive intake of yang foods e.g. meat, fish, root vegetables, salt, etc. This is an example of the ancient wisdom that the best course in life is 'moderation in all things'. Excess seems to bring about harmful imbalances.

The nose

The nose and the area just above and around the nose can give a lot of diagnostic indications.

- The area above the nose going up into the forehead tells us about the liver. A large smooth area here which has few or no creases shows that the person was born with a relatively yin liver this can indicate the likelihood of the liver being easily overwhelmed by toxins. It can also show a liking for yin substances (alcohol, sugar, drugs) and even a tendency to addiction.

- A yang liver is indicated by a well-defined central vertical line. There is a liking for strong flavours, yang foods and activities and a tendency to anger easily.

- If this area is very spotty or itchy it means the liver is not coping very well and this is probably due to an overload of sugar, fats, animal products, milk or cheese. Sometimes it can be that the liver is having to cope with alcohol, medical or recreational drugs.

- Traditionally, the area between the eyebrows should be free from hair. If the eyebrows meet in the middle this is considered a sign of extreme yang liver with possible difficulty controlling anger.

- Just below the eyebrows at the top of the nose there is sometimes a horizontal crease, this area relates to the pancreas. If this crease is present

'The nose and the area just above and around the nose can give a lot of diagnostic indications.'

the organ is overworked. Also the area can be red or appear puffy. Either of these extremes can mean a tendency to blood sugar problems like hypoglycaemia or diabetes and it is a good idea to watch the intake of carbohydrates and sugars. Remember that white sugar and white flour products can upset the blood sugar balance.

- The middle section of the nose, the bridge, is indicative of the stomach and if there is itchiness or redness in this area it shows that something you have eaten or drunk is irritating the stomach.

- The end of the nose is indicative of the heart and can give a lot of information about the state of this important organ.

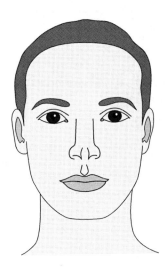

Pinched or bony tip of nose

Indicative of hardening of the arteries and poor heart function

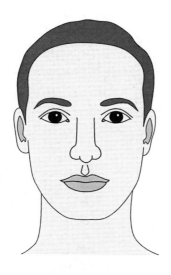

Bulbous nose

Indicative of an enlarged heart or circulatory disorders

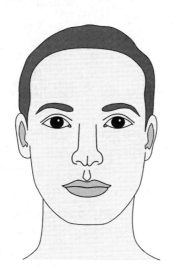

Cleft nose

Indicative of irregular heartbeat

In general:

- If the nose is swollen or the tip is hard a heart attack or stroke is possible.

- A red or purple nose can indicate hypertension/high blood pressure.

- Hairs growing out of the end of the nose (not nostril hairs) show that the heart is unhealthy and probably weakened by excessive intake of animal products or alcohol.

The cheeks

Large intestine

'Lung problems often show themselves in the cheeks particularly in the colour of this area.'

The large intestine is represented by the cheekbones. Swelling, redness or other discolouration can show problems with the bowels. Dry skin in this area or irritation, especially if there is a corresponding dryness of the lower lip, shows dehydration of the large intestine so it is advised you drink more water. If this area is often discoloured or sore, or if you have frequent bowel symptoms, seek medical advice.

Lungs

Lung problems often show themselves in the cheeks particularly in the colour of this area.

- Grey, often sunken cheeks are commonly seen where the lungs are weak or in the case of a chronic infection like tuberculosis. This is also the case with chronic lung damage such as emphysema or reduced lung capacity.

- Lung infections will often show as red cheeks.

- If the cheeks have a darker colour and are blotchey red or purple, this is a sign of problems with the blood supply in the lungs or damage caused by smoking, alcohol or other toxins.

The mouth

The top lip represents the stomach and the lower lip represents the intestines. For instance, a dry lower lip often coincides with dehydration of the large intestine that can cause constipation and headache. In this situation drinking lots of pure water will often solve the problem.

* Red lips represent inflammation.

* Dry lips show dehydration.

* Sore lips mean irritation.

* The corners of the mouth, where the upper and lower lips meet represents the place where the stomach and intestines meet i.e. the duodenum.

* Cracking in the corners of the mouth shows that the duodenum is under stress and if this becomes chronic it can show that a duodenal ulcer is starting.

The size of the lips can give some clues to the constitution of a person.

* A large (thick and fleshy) upper lip shows a good appetite and capacity of the stomach to hold or absorb food and drink.

* A thin upper lip shows the opposite.

* A large or thick lower lip especially if it is sore, red or bruised looking is indicative of inflammation or ulceration of the intestines.

* A narrow lower lip can indicate a smaller than usual or a tight large intestine. It is wise not to overload the digestive system in this case.

The area all around the mouth corresponds to the reproductive organs, hormonal balance, sexual energies and cycles.

* Any irritation, spots or unusual hair growth in this area can show hormonal changes.

* Often spots can appear in this area at ovulation, puberty or menopause.

* Prostate problems can show as skin blemishes in this area for older men.

The tongue

Different areas of the tongue traditionally show areas of the digestive system. The tongue can show changes more rapidly than they would appear on the face or other parts of the body

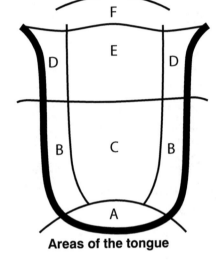

Areas of the tongue

'Different areas of the tongue traditionally show different areas of the digestive system.'

The areas of the tongue are as follows:

A – The last part of the digestive system, the descending colon and the rectum.

B – The large intestine.

C – The small intestine.

D – The duodenum, liver, gall bladder and pancreas.

E – The stomach.

F – The oesophagus.

Any soreness, ulceration, swelling or cracking on the tongue relates to the organ in the area that it occurs. The underside of the tongue is divided up in the same areas as the upper surface and is to do with the circulation of blood in the corresponding organs.

The colour of the upper surface of the tongue in the areas mentioned shows the following:

- Blue or purple – Too many yin foods i.e. sugars, fruits, juices, alcohol, drugs, medications.

- Red or dark red – Ulceration, inflammation.

- White – Poor circulation or stagnation of blood, mucus build-up, anaemia.

- White blotches – Excess animal fat or vegetable oil. Poor or overloaded digestion.

- Yellow – Liver and gall bladder are overloaded and causing problems in the area indicated. Also shows excessive production of bile, fat accumulations because of excess intake of animal fats, dairy products and eggs.

The colour of the underside of the tongue indicates the following:

- Purple – Lymph and blood vessel problems because of too many sugars, alcohol, drugs, medications or fruit.

- Red – Fluid build-up in the bloodstream (possibly leading to hypertension) from too many animal products, fruit, juices or liquid intake.

- Yellow – Build-up of fats and mucus due to a gall bladder problem or excess dairy products, eggs or poultry.

- Blue or bluey/green – Circulatory problems (possibly leading to clogging of the arteries) from over consuming animal fats, dairy products, or sugars and fruits.

On the following page there is an alternative chart showing a different interpretation of the areas of the tongue and the organs represented by them. This shows the diversity of ideas in oriental medicine.

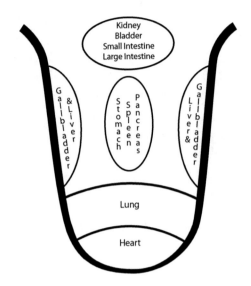

Pulse diagnosis

Pulse diagnosis is very popular amongst acupuncturists and is often the technique of choice amongst professional therapists.

It is, however, very complicated and difficult to learn. Some people say it can take a lifetime to learn completely. It is beyond the scope of a book like this, but suffice it to say that if a practitioner takes your pulses correctly and they have good training and intuition they will be able to glean a great deal of information from it.

Summing Up

- The face is a map and a helpful tool for diagnosing imbalances in the body. Insight as to the constitution and condition of a person may be gained by reading the face as well as other parts of the body.

- Imbalances in body systems or signs of poor health can often be identified by changes in colour or texture in different parts of the face or tongue.

- The forehead, ears, eyes, nose, cheeks, mouth and tongue all give indications as to general health and wellbeing.

- A further diagnostic aid in Oriental Diagnosis is to read the pulses. Specialised training and skill is required for this.

Chapter Three

Acupressure Today

Styles of acupressure

Many different styles of acupressure have developed over 5,000 or more years. There are therapies that use acupressure alone and some that use a combination of massage and acupressure. It is only natural that when therapies develop side by side over a long period of time there is a cross-fertilisation of ideas and techniques. This particularly happens when a therapy is taken to a new country or continent. It is thought that the Western form of massage, often termed 'Swedish massage', originally came from Asia. Along the way it has lost connection with ki and the energy systems, meridians and pressure points.

All the styles of acupressure are based on the principles of ki and its circulation throughout the body. Some work on the meridians and pressure points in a very specific way by applying pressure to the points directly, using finger, elbow or knuckle pressure. Sometimes shaped massage tools made from wood, stone or synthetic materials are used. Other styles use a more generalised massage technique, which, although less focused on specific points, encourages the flow of ki through the meridians. To a greater or lesser degree the various forms of acupressure also encourage the flow of lymphatic fluid (the body's drainage system), the circulation of blood and encourage relaxation of muscles.

To give an idea of the diverse applications of acupressure and the kinds of treatment commonly available, here is a more in depth look at some popular therapies.

'All the styles of acupressure are based on the principles of ki and its circulation throughout the body.'

Shiatsu

The Japanese word 'shi' means finger and 'atsu' means pressure. Shiatsu literally means 'finger pressure'. Shiatsu was developed from Anma in the early part of the 20th century in Japan. Now there are many variations on the original form of shiatsu but all are based on the same principles.

History

Tokujiro Namikoshi was born in 1905 on the Japanese island of Shikoku. At the age of 7 his family moved to the northern Island of Hokkaido, where the climate was harsher. His mother began to suffer aches and pains in her joints. Today she would have been diagnosed with rheumatoid arthritis. There was no medical help available and Namikoshi began stroking and pressing the parts of his mother's body that were painful. His mother was given relief by this, and he developed sensitivity and skill. Eventually his mother was cured of her condition and Namikoshi was inspired to study the human body. He went on to develop a technique based on thumb pressure which became Shiatsu. The first 'Shiatsu Institute of Therapy' was opened on Hokkaido in 1925 and in 1953 Shiatsu was taken to America by Sensei (Master or Teacher) Tokujiro Namikoshi and his son Toru. Since that time Shiatsu has become one of the most popular Acupressure based therapies and is practised in many parts of the world. Several varieties of Shiatsu have developed over the years and new ones undoubtedly continue to do so.

'Traditionally Shiatsu is given with the client lying on a futon mattress on the floor, through light clothing. In common with all acupressure treatments no massage oil is used.'

Traditionally, Shiatsu is given with the client lying on a futon mattress on the floor, although a massage couch can be used or if the client has difficulty lying down a massage chair might be more suitable. Often, shiatsu is given through light clothing although it can be applied to the skin. In common with all acupressure treatments no massage oil is used.

Shiatsu works on the 12 main meridians plus the Central and Governing Vessels, which are described in chapter 1. Charts showing the meridians in detail are shown in Part 2 of this book. There are over 300 pressure points (tsubo in Japanese) on these meridians that may be used in a Shiatsu treatment.

In shiatsu pressure points are stimulated in a variety of ways:

- The thumb or finger are used for focused pressure.

- Two fingers side by side are used for wider pressure points or to moderate the pressure.

- Where a point is small or in a tight spot the tip of the little finger or index finger may be used, for instance when treating Bladder 1 which is a pressure point in the corner of the eye socket near the nose.

- The elbow is used on fleshy areas like the buttocks, thighs or lower back.

- The knuckles can be used with a rocking movement down the side of the spine on the Bladder meridian.

Shiatsu also uses various stretching techniques where the practitioner gently supports parts of the client's body (arm, leg, shoulder, etc.) and gently twists and extends or stretches the limbs or torso. Percussion is used on muscular areas or on the upper back. This can be applied with cupped or flat hands or with the side of the fist or hand. Two hands can be used together to stretch or squeeze large muscles or groups of muscles.

Some of the techniques used to stimulate pressure points in shiatsu

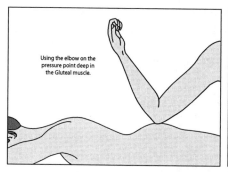

Using the elbow on the pressure point deep in the Gluteal muscle.

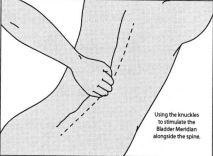

Using the knuckles to stimulate the Bladder Meridian alongside the spine.

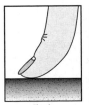
Thumb

Fingertip

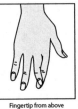
Fingertip from above

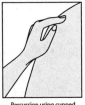
Percussion using cupped
hands on upper back
(alternating hands)

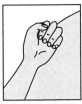
Percussion using the side
of the fist

Shiatsu treatments

'Ideally regular shiatsu sessions help maintain balance in the flow of ki throughout the body. This goes a long way towards supporting good health and vitality.'

A shiatsu session usually treats the whole person rather than a particular area or problem. Regular shiatsu maintains the balanced flow of ki, thereby supporting health and vitality. Having said that, shiatsu can be applied to specific areas for particular problems.

Examples are:

- Digestive, reproductive and bowel problems are helped by giving Ampuku therapy. This is a gentle method of working on the whole abdomen. It does not work on specific pressure points but instead generalised pressure using several fingers at once is applied to the abdomen. The pressure is applied slowly, gradually and as the client exhales. The hand moves from one adjacent area of the abdomen to the next in a clockwise direction. The first cycle is quite shallow and each time a circuit of the abdomen is completed the next is slightly deeper. This treatment enhances the flow of ki in the abdominal area and helps improve the blood flow and natural rhythmic movements of the small and large intestines (peristalsis). Ampuku is not to be applied after recent surgery, during pregnancy or if abdominal cancer has been diagnosed.

- Headache, nervous tension, hypertension and many back pains are often helped by giving neck shiatsu. One advantage of neck shiatsu is that the neck is very accessible and can be easily treated. Often I find that people who have never experienced any kind of massage or acupressure treatment before, and may be nervous about it, will allow a gentle neck treatment to take place. It is less invasive or strange to many people than someone working on their back or abdomen for instance. The neck is very sensitive and delicate and is always treated with great care and respect. Apart from the complicated bone structure (there are 7 neck vertebrae) and the vital nerves and blood vessels, there are many important meridians that run through the neck. Central and Governing Vessels, Bladder, Triple Heater, Stomach and Gall Bladder meridians can all be influenced during neck shiatsu.

- Foot shiatsu is in many ways similar to reflexology in that working on the feet can influence all parts of the body. If for some reason the whole body is not accessible for a full shiatsu treatment then giving foot shiatsu will still do a great deal of good to the whole system.

Seated Acupressure Massage

This relatively recent form of acupressure was born, like so many good things, at Apple Computers in Silicon Valley, California in 1984. David Palmer began giving 15-minute neck, back and shoulder treatments to employees at Apple. When he realised the popularity of these sessions he developed a special portable, folding massage chair.

The modern versions of the massage chair vary in construction, some are made from tubular metal. Others, like the one I use in my clinic, are made from wood. All are softly and hygienically upholstered. The client sits on the chair leaning forwards at a comfortable angle. There is a pad which supports the chest and a face support. The arms are supported in front of the body on an armrest. There are optional knee rests. All the supports are highly adjustable to accommodate all shapes and sizes of client.

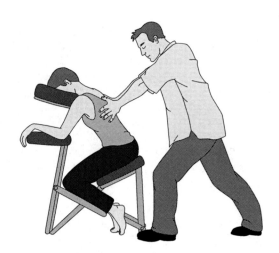

Seated Acupressure Massage

Seated Acupressure treatment

A basic Seated Acupressure Massage treatment is known as the Kata. 'Kata' is a term more often used in karate and other martial arts. It refers to a series of movements which are performed, almost like a dance.

In seated acupressure massage the Kata is usually a 15 to 20-minute routine of pressing, kneading, stretching and gentle tapping on the head, neck, shoulders and back. The Kata is performed in a specific order and the movements flow into one another in a smooth dancelike way. The techniques used are taken from Anma, one of the oldest acupressure systems, and over 60 pressure points are treated during the basic Kata. The Kata can be adapted to avoid areas where there may be an injury. Extra sequences may be added, for instance to the legs or face. The elbow, hand, thumbs, edge of hand, side of fist and fleshy part of the forearm are all used to work on the meridians and soft tissues.

The meridians that are worked on in the basic Kata (which includes the head, neck, shoulders and back) are: Small Intestine, Bladder, Gall Bladder, Large Intestine, Lung, Heart Protector, Triple Heater, Heart and Governing Vessel. Because all the meridians are connected in one large circuit by the internal meridians of the body, work on any part of the meridian system will affect all other parts to some extent. Extending the Kata to include the legs and feet would treat the rest of the meridians directly.

Aims of Seated Acupressure Massage

Seated Acupressure Massage works in a similar way to Anma and Shiatsu in that it aims to promote a healthy state by balancing the ki throughout the whole body. A session is shorter than the average Shiatsu or Anma session or indeed the average massage. If the client is used to a 45-minute treatment then a Seated Acupressure Massage session may at first seem short. Despite the fact that fewer pressure points are stimulated and the treatment is shorter, this form of acupressure can be just as effective. Clients will often comment that they feel 'invigorated and alert' after a session. Another comment that I often hear is that they feel 'relaxed yet alert'. I am often pleasantly surprised that even a five or ten-minute seated acupressure treatment, doing a condensed form of the Kata, can produce exciting results.

Seated Acupressure Massage came about originally as a treatment for the workplace, but because of the flexibility of using a portable chair and the fact that the client doesn't have to undress, it can be used virtually anywhere. Some of the places where it has been used are: airport lounges; cruise liners; music festivals; mind, body and spirit festivals; factories; offices; shopping centres; beaches; in health clinics and many more.

'Seated Acupressure Massage came about originally as a treatment for the workplace, but because of the flexibility of using a portable chair and the fact that the client doesn't have to undress it can be used virtually anywhere.'

> 'The underlying principle of applied kinesiology is that there is a relationship between the function of specific muscles, meridians, the lymphatic system and the rest of the mind/body.'

Case study

Soon after qualifying in Seated Acupressure Massage (in 1999), I was invited to take part in a Healing Fair in Birmingham, which was run by the college. We were offering ten minute 'taster' sessions so that people could experience an acupressure massage with little financial cost. The day was busy and the treatments were popular. About halfway through the day, a lady, who appeared to be in her mid-fifties, arrived in a wheelchair. She asked the person in charge if she would be able to have a treatment even though she had very limited mobility. He then asked me if I was prepared to treat this lady, and I agreed to do so.

With some help and support we managed to get her onto the chair and I asked her some standard questions about her health, etc. It transpired that in her twenties this lady had a very difficult labour and was eventually taken to the operating theatre for a caesarean. Tragically, as she was being transferred to the operating table from the trolley they dropped her and her back was broken. She had been disabled ever since and her mobility was getting worse.

I gave her the ten-minute treatment as requested. When I finished I asked how she felt. The lady said, 'Amazing,' then she reached up with her right hand and touched the top of her head. She said, 'I can't believe that, I haven't been able to brush my hair for thirty years.' On standing up and getting into the wheelchair she said, 'That was a lot easier and less painful too.'

Seated Acupressure Massage came about originally as a treatment for the workplace, but because of the flexibility of using a portable chair and the fact that the client doesn't have to undress it can be used virtually anywhere. Some of the places where it has been used are: airport lounges, cruise liners, music festivals, Mind, Body and Spirit Festivals, factories, offices, shopping centres, beaches, in health clinics and many more.

Applied Kinesiology – Touch for Health

Background

In 1964, Dr. George Goodheart, an American chiropractor, found a way of using mainstream medical kinesiological tests (muscle testing) to assess the function of meridians and body systems. This was the birth of Applied Kinesiology. Dr. John Thie (also a chiropractor) then devised a simplified version called 'Touch for Health' which was intended for use by laypeople.

Research and development of kinesiology is a continuous process and there are many versions/variants of kinesiology available today. The underlying principle is the same, that there is a relationship between the function of specific muscles, meridians, the lymphatic system and the rest of the mind/body. The various forms of kinesiology have different ways of testing using muscles to find imbalances and then using different modalities to rebalance them. The principle is that if the meridians and body systems are in a state of balance and harmony then optimal health can be enjoyed.

A typical session

What follows is a description of one way of working with Applied Kinesiology. This is the approach that I take in my own clinic. There are many other approaches and if you seek out a practitioner it is important that you ask them how they work and what kind of problems they treat.

I usually work with the client lying on their back on a massage couch or seated if they cannot lie down. I ask about any injuries or physical limitations in order to decide on the best method of testing to use. If the client has good mobility I will use a different test for each of the meridians. This involves placing the arms or legs in specific positions to isolate the muscle groups I want to test. I then ask the client to hold the position (i.e. resist) while I push gently and steadily. I then assess the strength of the muscle group and this gives an indication of the state of the particular meridian I am testing. If the meridian is weak or not working I will usually use pressure points to restore the flow of ki. I then move on to the next meridian in the sequence until all 14 channels have been rebalanced and the flow of ki is restored.

If the client has a problem with mobility or an injury that doesn't allow me to do the individual tests for each meridian I will choose what we call a 'Strong Indicator Muscle' (SIM). It is possible to test any meridian using a SIM by a process called 'challenging'. If the practitioner pushes against a SIM and when the client resists the muscle is strong we can proceed. The practitioner pushes the SIM and asks the client to resist, at the same time the practitioner touches a particular pressure point (depending on the meridian being challenged) and if there is a problem with the meridian being tested the SIM will weaken. If all is well with the flow of ki then the SIM will stay strong. This is then repeated using the same SIM but different points until all the meridians have been tested and, if necessary, rebalanced.

At the end of a Touch for Health or Applied Kinesiology session the person often feels very relaxed and reports a sense of wellbeing. Some people say that everything seems brighter or sharper. Some have a feeling of increased energy.

Applications of Applied Kinesiology

Because of the nature of this approach to Applied Kinesiology, it can have a beneficial effect on many different physical, mental or emotional problems. This is because the whole of the meridian system is being cleared and balanced. Other applications of Applied or Systemic Kinesiology are for food intolerances and allergies, phobias, anxiety, enhancing performance in sport, improving mental skills, resolving relationship problems, and many more.

Emotional Freedom Technique (EFT)

Background

This recent addition to the family of acupressure treatments is primarily aimed at psychological and emotional problems, yet has been found effective for pain and physical problems too. Emotional Freedom Technique (commonly known as EFT) was developed in the 1990s by Gary Craig. Originally trained as an engineer, and later working in insurance, Gary Craig always had an interest in self-development and achieving human potential. Eventually, he worked in this field and trained with Dr. Roger Callaghan, the originator of Thought Field Therapy. Dr Callaghan, a clinical psychologist, had become interested in using meridian-based therapy to work on emotional/psychological problems after studying Applied Kinesiology. Dr Callaghan discovered that each problem could be treated by tapping on a particular combination of pressure points (termed an algorhythm). The algorhythm for each type of problem (i.e. phobia, anxiety, compulsion, fear, etc.) being different.

Gary Craig discovered that there was a way of treating any problem with a universal algorhythm and in fact the combination of pressure points was not the crucial factor in treating a particular condition. From this discovery, EFT was born. One of the more advanced theories that has developed from EFT is that the intent of the practitioner and the way in which the practitioner and client interact is as important as the actual choice of pressure points.

Unlike most other types of acupressure there are only a limited number of points that are used in the original EFT process. As I discovered later, through my own research into EFT-based therapy, other points can be used effectively.

Pressure points used in EFT

On the following page are some illustrations showing points used in EFT. They are described in relation to anatomical landmarks to help you to find them as easily as possible. Points on the face are most easily found initially by looking in a mirror. You can use points on the left or right side of the body. It is better if you use the fingers of the hand on the side opposite the point. It is okay to do both sides at once or just left or right. It is recommended to use the fingertips of the index and middle finger together, this covers a larger area than one finger and gives a better chance of locating the right point.

- EB 'EyeBrow' – This point is at the end of the eyebrow nearest the nose.

- SE 'Side of the Eye' – This point is level with the outer corner of the eye just behind the bony structure that forms the orbit of the eye (not as far back as the temple but just over the bony ridge).

- UE 'Under the Eye' – This point is on the bony ridge under the eye (in line with the pupil when looking straight ahead).

- UN 'Under the Nose' – This point is between the nose and the upper lip on the vertical midline of the face.

- Ch 'Chin' – This point is situated between the lower lip and the tip of the chin (in a hollow) also on the vertical midline of the face.

- CB 'CollarBone' – At the base of the throat, at about the spot where a man would knot a tie, is a soft 'notch' at the top of the breastbone. Just 1" to the left or right of this and 1" down is a bony protuberance where the breastbone, collarbone and first rib all come together. This is the point to work on.

- BN 'Beneath Nipple' – On a man this is about 2 fingers' width below the nipple. On a woman the point is below the nipple at the point where the breast joins the chest.

- UA 'Under Arm' – Measure the width of one hand (across the biggest knuckles) from the armpit downwards. This point is on the side of the ribcage.

- Th 'Thumb point' – This point is located at the base of the thumbnail on the side furthest from the other fingers.

- IF 'Index Finger' – This point is located at the base of the index fingernail on the side nearest the thumb.

- MF 'Middle Finger' – This point is at the base of the middle fingernail on the side nearest the index finger.

- BF 'Baby or Little Finger' – This point is to be found at the base of the little fingernail at the side nearest to the other fingers.

- KC 'Karate Chop' – This is between the top of the wrist and the base of the little finger on the fleshy area at the side of the hand.

- Gamut Point – This is between the big knuckles of the ring and little fingers and about ½ an inch towards the wrist.

- Sore Spot – This is the sorest spot you can find (if there is one) on the upper chest area, between the breast and the collarbone roughly halfway between the breastbone and the armpit. If a sore spot is found at the beginning of a treatment it should be stimulated before going any further, while repeating a simple 'set up' phrase such as 'Even though I have this . . . problem/fear/ pain . . . . I fully and completely accept myself'. When the sore feeling has gone it is okay to proceed with the rest of the treatment.

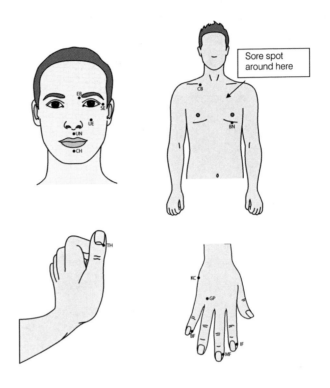

Sore spot around here

A basic EFT session (based on Gary Craig's original manual)

The EFT manual explains the basics of EFT, the techniques used and describes the location of the pressure points. It has always been freely available on Gary Craig's Emofree website. It is still widely available from many sources on the Internet. This availability obviously contributed hugely to the rapid growth of EFT and related therapies. Gary has always encouraged experimentation amongst experienced practitioners. Many people around the world learnt EFT by watching a series of very comprehensive CD video discs or DVDs. There are many courses available now with qualified instructors. Rather than try to explain the process I will give an example of an EFT treatment that I gave several years ago.

Case study

A middle aged farmer 'D' had a serious phobia regarding birds. I was treating him for an unrelated problem at the time and one day 'D' told me that he was contemplating a big change in his business and his life. He was planning to turn his farm over to free-range egg production. Then he told me about his fear of birds: 'I wondered if you can do anything about it with this new therapy you do?' He went on to explain that he couldn't even touch a dead bird without feeling really ill, let alone enter a building containing thousands of live birds.

The day came for 'D's' EFT session and we started by talking in depth about the background to his problem. This helped to bring the pattern of disrupted energies to the forefront of his energy system (meridians). This is a good start because EFT works by 'resetting' the disrupted energy patterns that have caused the emotional problem ('D's' phobia) in the first place.

I asked 'D' to vividly imagine himself going into a confined space containing a lot of hens. I then asked how he felt. 'Awful' was the reply. I asked how bad the fear was on a scale of one to ten. 'Eleven' he replied! I then started the process by checking 'D's' upper chest area to see if there was a 'sore spot'. I found a particularly sore area and got him to repeat the affirmation 'Even though I have this terrible fear of birds I fully and completely accept myself' while rubbing the spot. We repeated this three times and the place I was rubbing was no longer sore. This signified that the first part of the process was done.

Then I went straight into the next phase and started tapping each of the EFT tapping points about seven times in sequence. While I was tapping each point I said the 'reminder phrase' in this case 'This bird phobia'. 'D' repeated the phrase back to me on each occasion. When we completed all of the points I asked 'D' to imagine the scenario with the hens in the enclosed space again and to rate the level of fear on a scale of one to ten. 'Four' was the reply. 'Ok' I said 'tell me what exactly causes you to fear these birds'. 'It's the way they move, they're so unpredictable, and the feathers, they're horrible.' So we repeated the tapping on the sequence of points twice more. The first time using the reminder phrases 'These moving birds', 'These flapping birds', 'These unpredictable birds'. The next sequence the phrase was 'These horrible feathers'.

I then asked 'D' to imagine the scenario with the hens once more. This time his fear level was zero. So I said to him that I was sure his phobia had cleared and that he would be fine with birds and particularly with hens from that time on. At the time we were working at my home and there were quite a few hens in the area. It just so happened that as I was saying goodbye to 'D' and I opened the door, a large red hen was standing almost outside the door! I quickly reached down and picked her up. First I asked 'D' to stroke her and see how he felt, then I gave her to him to hold. He felt fine.

D now has a successful business involving looking after many thousands of free range hens.

Summing Up

- Over time many different styles of acupressure have developed.

- Some have become therapies in their own right.

- Popular acupressure-based treatments include shiatsu, seated acupressure massage and EFT.

- Each has their own unique style and cover a wide range of health issues from the physical to the emotional.

Chapter Four

Acupressure and Wellbeing

Common physical problems and how acupressure helps

Physical health problems fall into two categories: acute and chronic. Acute problems come on quickly, often without warning and may be something that you have only experienced rarely or never had before.

Acute or chronic?

Examples of acute health problems are: colds and flu, upset stomach, food poisoning, occasional constipation and diarrhoea, occasional headache, hangover, fever, muscular strain, sprains, fractures, stroke, heart attack, bruising, convulsions (especially febrile), vomiting, fainting, and so on.

Chronic health conditions include cancer, multiple sclerosis, CFS (chronic fatigue syndrome), Crohn's disease, colitis, irritable bowel, emphysema, recurrent migraine, fibromyalgia, chronic heart disease, diabetes, chronic circulatory problems, arthritis, rheumatoid arthritis, skin diseases, inherited problems of major organs and systems, asthma, and many more.

The way you would use acupressure to deal with a chronic problem may well differ from how you would approach an acute problem. An acute situation, like a simple headache or an upset stomach, would be approached from the point of view of simply treating the symptoms. Problems associated with a chronic illness would take into account the underlying causes to a greater extent when choosing the treatment.

Traditional or modern?

If you were to consult a practitioner, depending on which therapy you chose, they would assess and treat you accordingly. As you may well have realised by now the assessment or diagnosis is an important part especially in the more traditional therapies like Anma and Shiatsu. With a relatively new therapy like Seated Acupressure Massage the approach is very much that whatever the problem is the treatment simply aims to improve the flow of ki and the overall energy levels. The point being that the whole person (physical, mental and emotional) should then be more able to cope with the symptoms or problems, and healing can begin.

To self-treat or not?

When using acupressure for yourself, unless you have undergone training in a particular therapy, your approach will be mostly symptom treatment. It must be said at this point if you experience any symptom or problem that you don't recognise as a very simple problem, or if any symptom persists, becomes frequent or a regular problem, consult your doctor.

Acupressure is not a replacement for Western medicine and is not intended as a treatment for serious medical conditions. You can't stop a heart attack or a stroke with acupressure, or mend a broken leg. If you have a hangover, a cold, or arthritis – it can be invaluable in easing your discomfort.

'Acupressure is not a replacement for Western medicine and is not intended as a treatment for serious medical conditions. You can't stop a heart attack or a stroke with acupressure, or mend a broken leg. If you have a hangover, a cold, or arthritis – it can be invaluable in easing your discomfort.'

Mental or emotional problems and how acupressure helps

The way that you might approach mental or emotional problems depends very much on the severity of the problem. If you need dental treatment but have a fear of going to the dentist or have a problem with public speaking and you have to give a presentation then self-help is fine. If you can't leave the house because of agoraphobia or have some serious obsession or depression then it is time to seek help from a medical practitioner. If you are in doubt talk to a health professional.

Help with common anxieties

Therapies such as TFT, EFT and their variants can be very helpful for a great many of the everyday anxieties, phobias and confidence issues that seem so common now, in our hectic and high pressure world. They are also effective at enhancing performance in sports, performing arts, sales, exams, and many other areas of life. Often this is due to the process of removing self-doubt and fear of failure. Sometimes it is simply getting the 'self' out of the way and just allowing things to happen.

Change of attitude or perspective

Often people get in the habit of catastrophising and imagining the worst. This is the 'but what if' approach to life rather than the 'if it arises I will deal with it' method. There are times when these types of therapy can change the perspective of a person and set them free.

'Therapies such as TFT, EFT and their variants can be very helpful for a great many of the everyday anxieties, phobias and confidence issues that seem so common now, in our hectic and high pressure world.'

Case Study

A lady in her forties ('C') had been undergoing treatment for some time for stress related back pain and tension. A time came when she had to move house. This meant that she would have to travel further for her appointments and she was worried about the driving. When asked to explain more about this problem, it turned out that she became fearful and lacked confidence when on dual carriageways, motorways and busy roads in general. Busy roundabouts were a big problem to her.

I asked 'C' if she would like to try an EFT session to deal with this fear and anxiety. At first she was quite sceptical and so I said I would give her a session at no extra charge after her normal treatment. 'C' agreed and the next time I saw her we did the EFT. Because I had already balanced 'C's' meridians during her normal session it meant that we could shorten the EFT process somewhat. I asked 'C' to vividly imagine the most recent situation where she had felt fear and anxiety when driving. Then I got her to repeat suitable phrases whilst tapping a sequence of pressure points. After the first round of pressure points I asked her to visualise the fearful driving situation. She had great difficulty visualising it fully, which I always take as a good sign.

'C' went home and the next time I saw her she told me that not only had she been able to drive without the usual problems but she had much more confidence dealing with difficult situations at work and home!

This is a common outcome, when treating a specific fear, other fears may become less of a problem.

Years later the driving anxieties have not returned.

Helping the effects of shock

Often there are difficult situations in life which arise suddenly or unexpectedly: arguments, confrontations, illness, bereavement, accidents, aggression, indecision, being overwhelmed (to name but a few). These situations can very often be helped by something as simple as becoming aware of your breathing and regulating it, feeling your feet firmly on the ground or using one or two pressure points. Some knowledge of acupressure, EFT or TFT can be invaluable in enabling you to deal with such difficulties.

Self-help

Part 2 of this book is in the form of a self-help manual and there are many useful pressure points and simple techniques that you can use (often with no one else noticing – very handy in, for instance, an interview).

Fingertip tapping

I have often used a simple EFT technique that I devised to deal with situations I found stressful. Here is a good example that occurred a few years ago.

I had been writing poetry and short stories for a few years when a friend told me that my local town was having a literary festival. As part of this festival he explained that there was to be an 'open mike' poetry night for poets to come along and read their work. Immediately I said I would do it. The night came along and I had several poems ready to read out. So I sat down and had a beer while waiting my turn.

Very gradually, I began to feel nervous, for no obvious reason. I felt good about the poetry I had written, I had taught and given talks to groups and given demonstrations of my therapies. Nevertheless I felt shaky and a bit wobbly inside. So, I decided to try a dose of my own medicine. A year or two earlier I had devised a very simple way of using EFT which involves tapping the fingertips together while repeating a suitable phrase or affirmation.

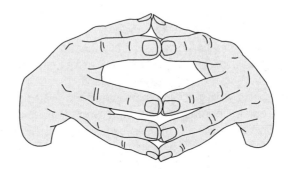

Fingertip tapping

This technique has the advantage of being easy to use without anyone noticing (Gary Craig, the founder of EFT, called it 'Secret Tapping' when I told him about it). So I was tapping away under the table and saying, 'Even though I feel nervous about this performance, and I don't know why! I completely accept myself.' When the time came to go on stage, I was calm and collected and read out my poems without a single wobble!

Prevention is better than cure

'One of the main principles of natural or holistic healing is that ill health often comes about because of a weakening of the body's defences or an imbalance of some kind in a particular body system.

The immune system

Have you ever wondered why one person in a family will get an infection but another doesn't? Or why, when a supposedly highly infectious virus, like 'bird flu', is around not everybody succumbs to it? The holistic explanation is that one person will have an immune system that is more healthy and quick to 'learn' to fight a new virus than another. There are lots of ideas as to why this is. Many people believe that the massive rise of synthetic chemicals in the environment and in our food, overuse of chemical drugs and antibiotics, exposure to things like mobile phones and electromagnetic fields and de-natured 'junk foods' all weaken the immune system. There is no doubt that we have far more of these things to deal with than at any other time in our history.

'One of the
main principles
of natural or
holistic healing
is that ill health
often comes
about because
of a weakening
of the body's
defenses or
an imbalance
of some kind
in a particular
body system.'

64

Further considerations

I add another layer to this idea and say that all these things have a negative effect on the energy system of living beings. They can cause imbalance in the meridians and lower ki. As well as the factors mentioned, ki levels can be adversely affected by mental and emotional stress, particularly unresolved or ongoing stresses, shock, physical trauma and even things like sudden changes of environment. A good example is thermal shock. If a person goes suddenly from a warm environment to a much colder one, without the right clothing or preparation they will often become unwell. This is due to the meridians being unable to quickly adjust to the rapid temperature change. Yet with the right training it is said that a person can control their ki to the extent that they can sit on the ground in freezing conditions, wearing very light clothing and melt the snow around them.

Regular work to balance the meridians and maintain ki, whether it is through having acupressure therapy or practising tai chi, chi gong or yoga, may not give you the ability to melt snow, however it may help to keep you more healthy and happy. Anything that we can do to maintain optimum health and prevent problems taking hold has to be better than taking desperate measures when things have started to go wrong. I have included some simple daily routines in the second half of this book that help maintain a healthy equilibrium.

Individual equilibrium

A healthy equilibrium will vary from one person to another and will be unique to them. Depending upon an individual's constitution, inherited factors, lifestyle and environment, the level of health achievable will vary.

'Ki levels can be adversely affected by mental and emotional stress, particularly unresolved or ongoing stresses, shock, physical trauma and even things like sudden changes of environment.'

Summing Up

- Physical health problems fall into two categories: acute and chronic. Though each may require a different approach, both will lower one's energy.

- Some acupressure treatments aim simply to improve the flow of ki and overall energy levels. Others have a more targeted approach, focusing on specific problems.

- A change in attitude can often shift common anxieties.

- Fingertip tapping is a most useful self-help tool especially in emotionally charged situations.

- Levels of ki are often affected by mental, emotional, spiritual or environmental stresses.

- Unresolved or ongoing problems disrupt the flow of ki throughout the body.

Part 2

Chapter Five

Understanding the Body

This chapter is intended to give a basic understanding of how the human body is put together (anatomy) and how it works (physiology). The aim is that I, the writer, and you, the reader, have some common terminology and understanding of what the bits and pieces that make up our bodies are called and how to locate them. This is simply to avoid confusion. Often I have had a client say they have a 'stomach pain' only to find later that they don't have a pain in their stomach (high in the abdomen and just below the ribcage) but they have pain in their lower abdomen often caused by the large intestine or period pain. Another area of confusion is that people talk about their hips (the joint at the top of the upper leg) when they mean the crest of the pelvis (the bony bit that sticks out at the bottom of the waist).

'The joints are particularly useful landmarks when finding your way around the body.'

The section on anatomy has the bare essentials to act as a reference when explaining where pressure points are located. Likewise, the physiology section is kept simple but will give sufficient information to help understand what is going on in the body when symptoms arise. This enables you to decide how to deal with them or to describe your problem to a practitioner or doctor.

Basic anatomy

The skeleton

Let's start with the skeleton. I will often refer to bones when describing where to find a pressure point. The joints are particularly useful landmarks when finding your way around the body. Layman's names for bones and joints will be used unless there is a good reason to do otherwise. The diagrams are labelled with the names that will be used in the following chapters.

One of the criteria for choosing pressure points for self-help in this book is that they should be easy to find and to use. Included are diagrams of the location of bones, joints and muscles that will help with the location of the pressure points that are mentioned later.

Human skeleton

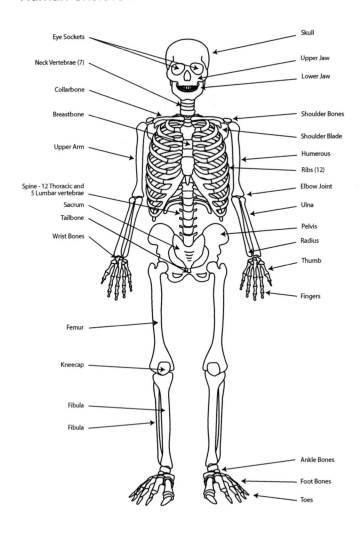

Eye Sockets

Neck Vertebrae (7)

Collarbone

Breastbone

Upper Arm

Spine - 12 Thoracic and 5 Lumbar vertebrae

Sacrum

Tailbone

Wrist Bones

Femur

Kneecap

Fibula

Fibula

Skull

Upper Jaw

Lower Jaw

Shoulder Bones

Shoulder Blade

Humerous

Ribs (12)

Elbow Joint

Ulna

Pelvis

Radius

Thumb

Fingers

Ankle Bones

Foot Bones

Toes

The hand

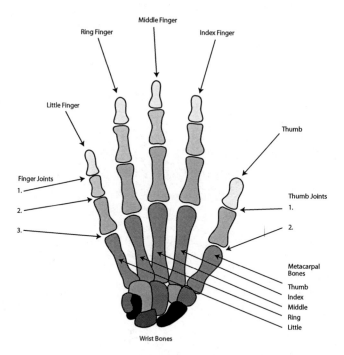

Middle Finger

Ring Finger

Index Finger

Little Finger

Thumb

Finger Joints
1.
2.
3.

Thumb Joints
1.
2.

Metacarpal
Bones

Thumb
Index
Middle
Ring
Little

Wrist Bones

The foot

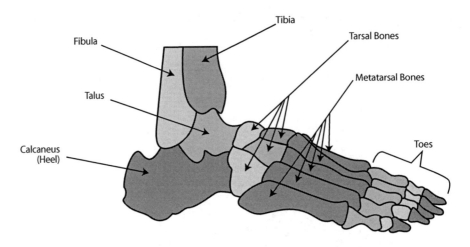

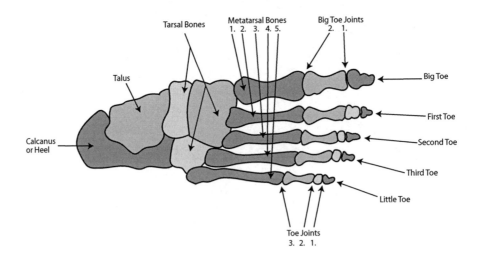

Muscles

Mostly common names are used, and only major muscle groups are shown for reference.

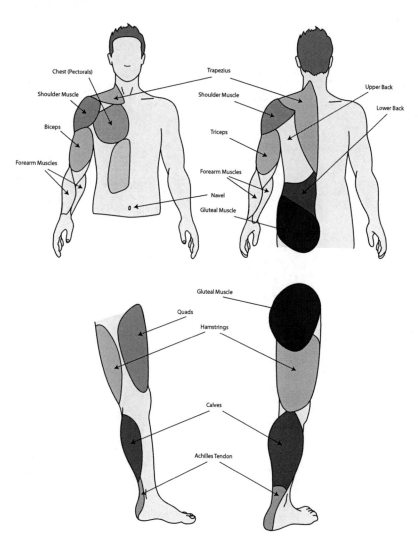

Basic physiology

The human body is incredibly complex and this section does not attempt to explain its workings in any great detail. It will attempt to give some basic knowledge of the organs and systems of the body and what they do.

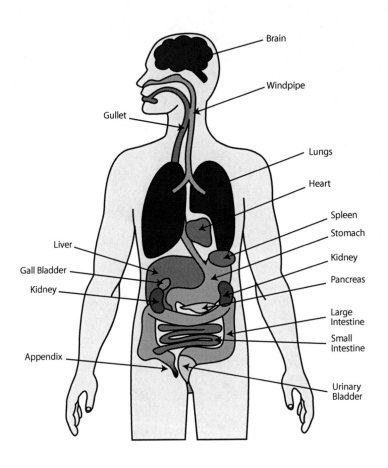

Main organs

On the previous page is a simplified diagram of the main organs of the human body. The functions of the organs are listed below.

- Brain – Thought occurs in the brain as well as control of the automatic processes of the body, for instance breathing, heart function, blood pressure, balance and much more. Special organs in the brain (pituitary, pineal and hypothalamus) control appetite, body clock and temperature, hormones and metabolism (energy release and storage of fat).

- Lungs – The lungs remove waste gasses (mostly carbon dioxide) from the red blood cells and take in oxygen from the air which is absorbed by the red blood cells and transported around the body.

- Heart – The heart is a complicated pump and does two jobs at once. One half of the heart pumps blood to the lungs where carbon dioxide is removed and fresh oxygen is absorbed. The oxygenated blood then returns to the heart. The other half of the heart then pumps the blood around the body delivering oxygen and nutrients to the tissues and organs and collecting waste products and carbon dioxide.

- Stomach – The stomach is where food is sterilised with acid to kill any dangerous bacteria or other organisms. Full digestion starts in the stomach and some nutrients are absorbed.

- Small intestine – Digestion continues in the small intestine and different nutrients are processed and absorbed in different parts as the food travels through. The small intestine is around 23 feet long and contains many types of friendly bacteria that aid digestion.

- Large intestine – Once food passes from the small into the large intestine most of the absorption of nutrients has finished, although water, minerals, B vitamins and vitamin K are still absorbed in the large intestine. Waste matter passes out of the body via the rectum and anus.

- Spleen – The spleen recycles worn out red blood cells and acts as a reservoir for all kinds of blood cells. Lymphocytes, white blood cells, that are an important part of the immune system are produced in the spleen.

- Kidneys – The kidneys regulate the levels of essential chemicals in the bloodstream and remove toxins which are excreted as urine. They also have a role in controlling blood pressure.

- Pancreas – The pancreas releases enzymes which enable the body to digest carbohydrates and sugars. The other function of the pancreas is to release the enzyme insulin into the blood so that it can interact with glucose in the body to provide energy.

- Liver – The liver is the chemical factory of the body. It has hundreds of different functions. The liver manufactures proteins to repair the body and chemicals which are used for digestion. It stores glycogen which can be released into the bloodstream when the body has an urgent need for energy. The other major function is detoxifying the blood.

- Gall bladder – The waste product of the liver, bile, is collected in the gall bladder. When fatty or oily food is taken into the digestive system, as it reaches the small intestine the gall bladder squirts bile into the small intestine where it mixes with the food. This breaks down the fats and makes them a lot easier to digest.

Summing Up

▨ Having a very basic understanding of how the body is put together and how it works is most useful.

▨ The recognition of physical landmarks contributes to locating pressure points more easily.

▨ It is good to have some insight into the workings of some major organs.

Chapter Six

Meridians, Points and Techniques

The fourteen main meridians and vessels

There are twelve main meridians recognised in the West and, along with the Central and Governing Vessels, they comprise the fourteen main channels of energy used in acupressure. Some pressure points do not lie on these fourteen channels. There are other channels, including the internal meridians, which connect the surface meridians and vessels. This creates one continuous circuit of ki throughout the body and links with the universal ki.

In this chapter the location of the main meridians and vessels on the front and back of the body, and on the head and face, are illustrated. In the next chapter the location of the points are shown.

The charts that follow will give a good indication of where the meridians and vessels are to be found.

'There are twelve main meridians recognised in the West and, along with the Central and Governing Vessels, they comprise the fourteen main channels of energy used in acupressure.'

Meridians of the head and face

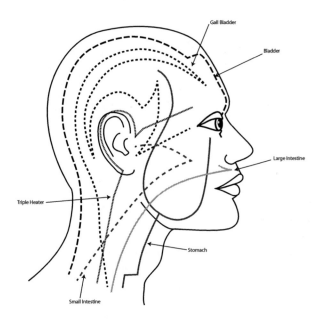

As well as the meridians shown above, the Central Vessel starts between the legs on the perineum and goes straight up the middle of the body finishing on the bottom lip. The Governing Vessel starts on the tip of the tail bone, goes up the centre of the spine and continues over the back and top of the head and down the centre of the face to the top lip.

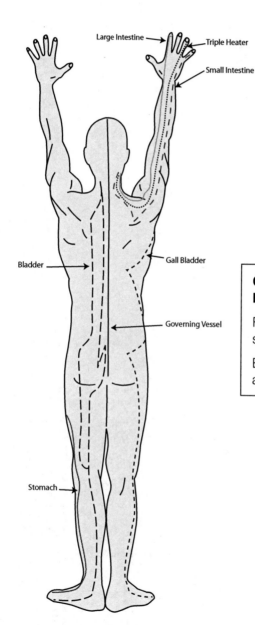

Large Intestine

Triple Heater

Small Intestine

Bladder

Gall Bladder

Governing Vessel

Stomach

Channels on the back of the Body

For clarity the channels are only shown on either the left or right.

Each Meridian exists to the left and right sides of the centre line.

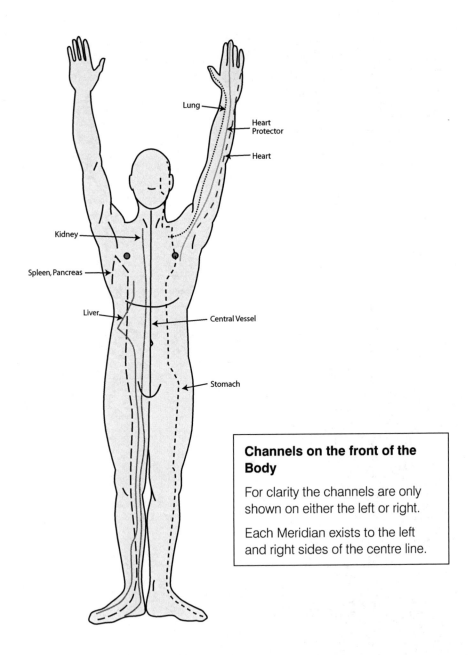

Lung

Heart
Protector

Heart

Kidney

Spleen, Pancreas

Liver

Central Vessel

Stomach

Channels on the front of the Body

For clarity the channels are only shown on either the left or right.

Each Meridian exists to the left and right sides of the centre line.

Finding pressure points

Charts showing meridians and pressure points are like maps. They can only give a guide to where things are. In fact they aren't quite as good as maps. Roads and mountains, villages and valleys don't move. A meridian chart is only true for an idealised, average human being. Humans vary greatly in size and shape as well as proportions of head, torso and limbs. So the charts can only ever be a guide.

In acupressure we use the proportions of the body of the person being worked on. So we use measurements of parts of the body to define where a pressure point is. The most commonly used measurements are one hand's width and one thumb's width. If you are working on your own body then use your hand or thumb. If you are working on someone else then use their hand or thumb size as a guide. Hand width is across the knuckles at the base of the fingers. Thumb width is across the knuckle.

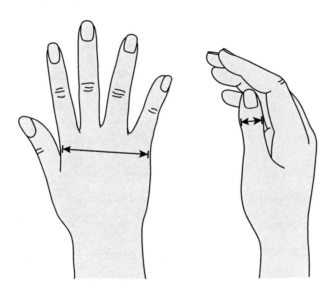

Example

There is a pressure point on the Triple Heater meridian which is very useful for pain in the arms, shoulders or ribs. It is also useful in an asthma attack. The point is one hand's width above the most obvious crease on the upper wrist, the same side as the back of the hand and in line with the middle finger. To locate the point:

- Find the crease on the wrist.

- Place your other hand so that the knuckle at the base of the little finger is against the crease, in line with the middle finger.

- The knuckle at the base of the first finger will then be next to the point.

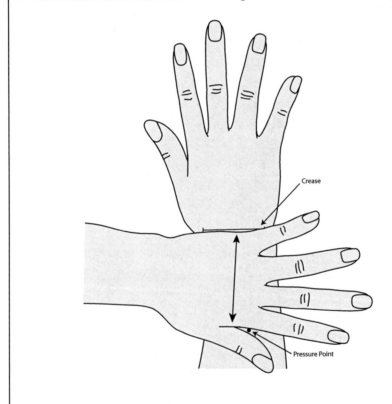

Crease

Pressure Point

Even using the charts and making measurements with thumb and hand width, it is necessary to use some intuition and sensitivity to find the exact pressure point. Often a pressure point is felt as a little depression in the skin/flesh. I have heard practitioners and teachers say that when feeling for a point your finger will fall into it.

What a pressure point feels like

When finding a pressure point on your own body, once you are as close as you can get with the aid of charts and descriptions, the final test is that a pressure point will be the most sensitive spot in that area. Again, with experience, you will recognise the feeling when you press on a point; it is like pain, but not pain. It is not usually an unpleasant feeling although it can be quite intense. Some points will always feel more sensitive than others and a few are painful. For instance Kidney 1, a point on the sole of the foot, is not a comfortable point to press. You will certainly know when you have found it! When the Kidney meridian is out of balance and this point needs attention, it can be sore to the slightest pressure.

In Japanese traditions a tsubo (pressure point) is commonly compared to a well. Like a well it can be empty or full. This is something that becomes noticeable with practice. Whether you press a point on yourself or someone else, you become aware that sometimes the finger sinks into the point easily and sometimes there is a resistance. If it feels 'full' i.e. there is resistance, you will want to maintain the finger pressure for a little longer.

Technique

Once you have found the pressure point the finger, thumb, elbow, or in some cases tool, rests gently on it. Pressure is then gradually increased, held for a few seconds and then released. If you are sensitive you will feel the finger or thumb sinking into the tsubo and then stopping as it reaches the bottom. The pressure is released more quickly than it was applied but it should be gentle, not sudden.

'Often a pressure point is felt as a little depression in the skin/flesh.'

Often it is recommended to gently rotate the finger in the tsubo, or vibrate it as pressure is applied. Occasionally it is necessary to repeat the pressure several times. A period of time (minimum of twenty minutes) is normally left before repeating treatment of a point or points.

How to press

More often than not, the tip of the thumb is used to apply pressure to a point. Partly this is because of the strength of the thumbs, compared to the other fingers. Other fingertips can be used if the angle is awkward or space is limited. The elbow and one or more knuckles can sometimes be employed.

Good examples are:

- When applying pressure to the first point of the Bladder meridian, between the nose and the tear duct of the eye (in the depression) where space is very limited, the tip of the little finger can be used.

- When applying pressure to points on the back, alongside the spine or on the top of the shoulders the elbow is very useful – see illustration.

- For the tiny points on the fingers, at the base of the fingernail, a blunt matchstick works well.

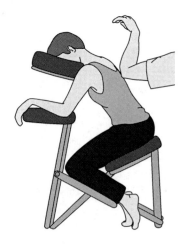

Using the elbow

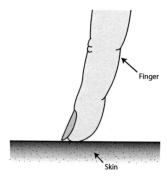

Finger

Skin

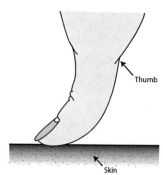

Thumb

Skin

The correct way to apply pressure with the finger, thumb and a matchstick.

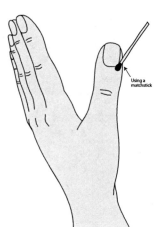

Using a matchstick

Summing Up

- Pressure points on 12 meridians and 2 vessels are used in acupressure.

- Charts are only a guide. Locating pressure points comes with practice.

- Usually the thumb is used to apply pressure, however other fingertips, knuckles or the elbow may be employed.

Chapter Seven

Pressure Points and Their Uses

Types of treatment

Acupressure can be used as a method of symptom relief in acute situations or as a means of support in a long-term or chronic illness. The approach to treatment is slightly different in these two situations.

Acute problems

This may be a situation such as an injury, a physical or emotional shock, an acute illness (like flu or stomach bug) or pain after dental treatment. In this case the acupressure can be used to ease symptoms, to deal with fear or panic or to relieve pain. Pressure points will be stimulated at intervals until the problem has resolved, for instance until recovery from the illness, shock or injury.

Chronic problems

A person may be suffering from a chronic, long-term illness or disability which involves physical or other symptoms like joint pain, headaches, nausea or dizziness. Acupressure can help in this sort of situation by using points on a daily basis as part of a routine to improve health and control symptoms. If the underlying problem is known and the symptoms are recognised as a part of the problem then acupressure may be valuable as an adjunct to other treatments or pain relief. Always speak to a doctor in these circumstances and get their approval.

'Acupressure can be used as a method of symptom relief in acute situations or as a means of support in a long-term or chronic illness.'

Recommended pressure points

The points recommended in this chapter are all traditional pressure points with a long history of effective use. They are chosen for the following reasons:

- Location – points will be easy to find.
- Easy to stimulate on one's own body.
- Effectiveness.
- Useful for common problems.
- Safety.

None of the points recommended could cause any adverse reaction or problem if they were to be used out of context. If a point recommended for one problem was mistakenly used for something else it could not do any harm. It would just be ineffective.

'Never use a pressure point where the skin is broken or damaged or where there is swelling or bruising.'

Safety and common sense

- If you are pregnant or think you may be pregnant, especially in the first three to four months, ask medical advice before using acupressure or any other kind of treatment.
- Never use a pressure point where the skin is broken or damaged or where there is swelling or bruising.
- Do not press on any delicate or vulnerable part of your own or another person's body, especially the eyes, in the ears, inside the nose or mouth, breasts, genitals or anus. No pressure points are recommended in this book on any of those areas.
- Do not try to substitute acupressure for serious medical attention. If you have any symptom that persists, gets worse, or that you don't recognise seek medical assistance.

Points, locations and uses

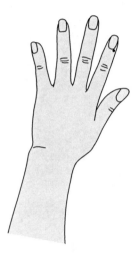

Large Intestine #1

Location:

Just below the corner of the nail on the index finger of both hands. Press with tip of thumbnail, a blunt matchstick or similar object for about 20 seconds; press on both hands.

Uses:

- Fever.
- Diarrhoea.
- Laryngitis.
- Pain in lower jaw.
- Toothache.
- During dental work.

Large Intestine #4

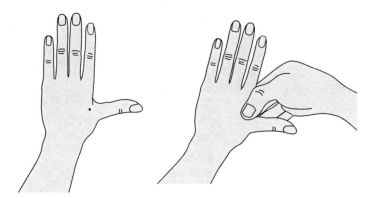

Location:

On the web of flesh between the thumb and hand, feel for the most sensitive spot in the middle of this fleshy area. If using this point on someone else, ask them to tell you when you are pressing on a sensitive spot. Place the pads of the index and middle fingers on the palm side of the area and press with the thumb for around 20 seconds gently rotating the thumb in tiny circles. Press the point on both hands.

Uses:

- Hangover symptoms.

- Headaches (especially if there are bowel symptoms like constipation or bloating).

- Lung problems including simple coughs and minor infections. If the problem gets worse or continues, consult a doctor.

- Facial tension.

- Chronic large intestine problems.

- Hot flushes.

- Traditionally this point is used for pain anywhere in the upper body, above the navel.

Large Intestine #20

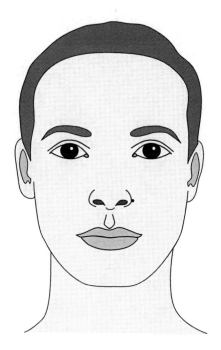

Location:

In the groove next to the side of the fleshy part of the nose on both sides, the point is just above the root of the canine tooth. Press firmly with the tip of the index finger for 20 seconds on each side.

Uses:

- Relieves blocked nose and sinuses.
- Helps to stop a runny nose.

In Do

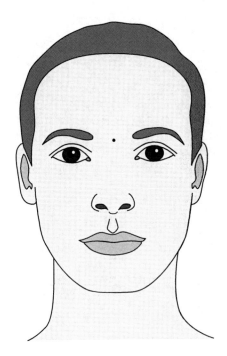

Location:

On the centre line of the face, between the eyebrows, press with thumb or fingertip for 15 to 20 seconds.

Uses:

- Sinus pain or congestion.
- Nasal blockage.
- Hot flushes.
- Headaches.

Stomach #3

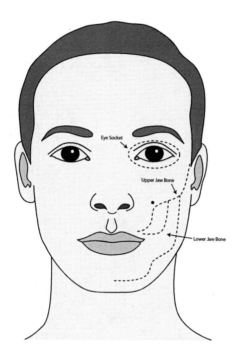

Location:

Directly below the eye, on the upper jaw bone below the level of the cheek bone. Looking in a mirror the point is almost directly below the pupil of the eye. Press with fingertip for 20 seconds on both sides. Also may be tapped rhythmically 7 to 14 times.

Uses:

- Fear (tap both sides).
- Sinus pain or blockage.
- Neuralgia of face.

Bladder #1

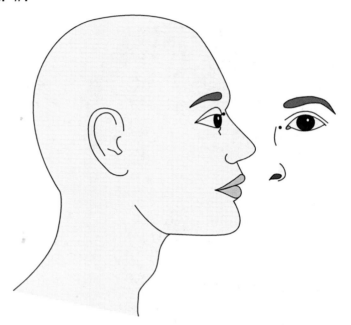

Location:

Between the tear duct and the nose at the inner corner of the eye. The point is located in a small depression. Press for 15 seconds with the tip of the little finger. Make sure that the fingernail is cut short and take extra care to avoid the eye itself. Press both sides.

Uses:

- Sore eyes.
- Puffy eyes.
- Tired eyes.
- Nose bleeds (seek medical help if the nose bleed continues or recurs).
- Traditionally, these points are stimulated daily by pinching and massaging with the thumb and finger, simultaneously on both sides, to improve vision.

Kidney #3

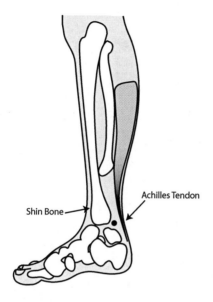

Achilles Tendon

Shin Bone

Location:

In the hollow between the ankle bone and the achilles tendon on both legs. Increase pressure gently, this point is often tender. Maintain pressure for 20 seconds. Avoid during pregnancy.

Uses:

- May help male sexual dysfunction.

- Traditionally used to support chronic kidney problems or weak kidney function.

Heart Protector #6 and #8

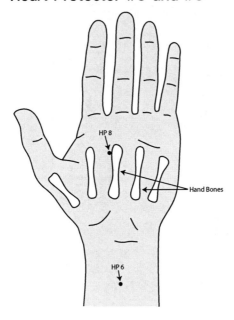

Location:

Heart Protector #6 can be found on the centre line of the inside of the wrist, in line with the middle finger, two thumbs' width from the most prominent line on the inner wrist. Press for 20 seconds on both arms with thumb tip.

Uses:

- Nausea.
- Vomiting.
- Palpitations.
- Motion sickness.

Location:

Heart Protector #8 is close to the middle of the palm of the hand. It is close to the top end of the middle metacarpal (hand) bone, as illustrated. There is a distinctive sensation when you press on this point, very different from the surrounding area. Press both hands with thumb tip for 7-10 seconds every 20 minutes until relief is felt. Use the first and middle finger on the back of the hand for support, similar to Large Intestine #4.

Uses:

* Anxiety.

* Exhaustion.

Heart Protector #9

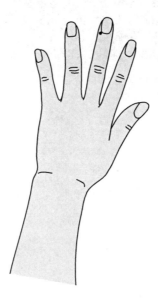

Location:

Just below the corner of the fingernail, towards the ring finger and little finger, on both hands. Press with tip of thumbnail, a blunt matchstick or similar for 20 seconds.

Uses:

- Menstrual pain and cramps.

- Anxiety.

- To regulate high or low blood pressure.

- Before dental work.

Lung #10

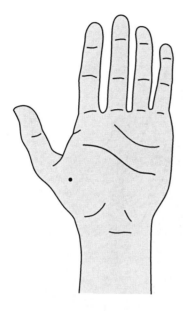

Location:

In the middle of the fleshy area at the base of the thumb. Press with the thumb tip while supporting the other side with the first and middle fingers (see Large Intestine #4). Press both hands for 20 seconds.

Uses:

- Coughing.
- Sore throat.
- Loss of voice.

Lung #11

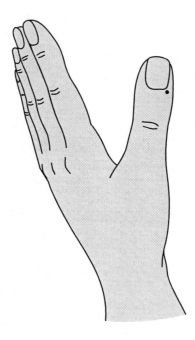

Location:

Just below the outer corner of the thumbnail. Press with thumbnail tip of the other hand or a blunt matchstick for 15 to 20 seconds.

Uses:

- Coughs.
- Sore throat.
- Pharyngitis.
- Tired arms and hands.

Lung #5

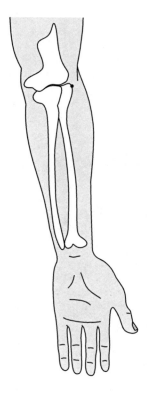

Location:

The point is on the crease of the elbow when the arm is bent. It is on the same side as the thumb and with firm pressure you will be able to feel the edge of the bone.

Uses:

- Respiratory allergies (hay fever or allergic asthma).
- Bronchitis.
- Helpful for giving up smoking.

Central Vessel #15 and #17

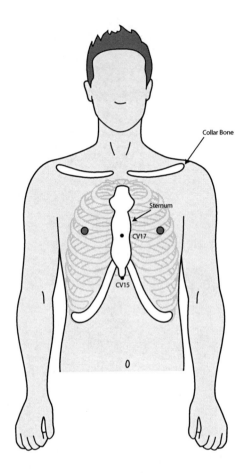

CV #15 location:

The point is located at the tip of the lower end of the sternum or breastbone on the centre line of the body. There is a distinct sensation when you press on the point, not painful, but not comfortable either. Press with a finger or thumb tip for 15 seconds.

Uses:

- Nausea.
- Seasickness.
- Hiccups.
- To boost energy.

CV #17

Location:

In the centre of the sternum, one hand's width down from the notch at the top of the sternum, level with the nipples on an adult male. Press with finger or thumb tip for 15 seconds.

Uses:

- Hiccups.
- Asthma.
- Raised blood pressure.
- Promotes lactation where there is a lack of milk.
- Hot flushes.
- Tender/sore breasts associated with menstrual cycle.

Spleen #6 and #9

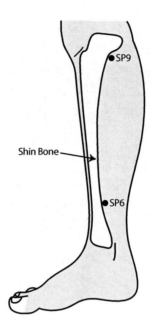

Spleen #6 location:

One hand's width above the top of the ankle bone, on the inside of the leg, just behind the shin bone. Press for 15 to 20 seconds on both legs.

Uses:

- Insomnia.

- Obesity.

- Digestive problems.

- Menstrual pains/cramps.

- Female reproductive or sexual problems.

- This point is called Leg Triple Yin. It is where the three yin leg meridians cross. A very powerful point for all 'female' problems or yin imbalances.

Spleen #9

Location:

In the hollow just below the knee joint on the inside of the leg, just behind the shin bone and below the head of the shin bone. Press for 20 seconds on both legs.

Use:

This is an energy release point for exhaustion. It is called the Ten Mile Point, because traditionally it allows you to walk an extra ten miles.

Liver #1 and #2

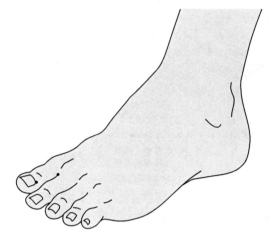

Liver #1

Location:

Just below the corner of the big toenail on the side adjacent to the other toes. Press with a blunt matchstick for 15 seconds on both big toes. If this is too uncomfortable or sensitive use your fingertip.

Uses:

- Abdominal discomfort.
- Constipation.
- Genitourinary problems e.g.cystitis. (This is not a substitute for medical attention).
- Pain in genitals e.g. bruised testicles after injury (consult your doctor).
- Difficulty passing urine when there is a painful urge to do so (consult your doctor).

Note: The last three points on this list are for temporary relief until you can get medical attention.

Liver #2 location:

On the web of skin between the joints at the base of the big and first toes, press firmly for 7 to 10 seconds with a slight circular motion. Press both feet. Repeat after 20 minutes if symptoms are slow in going.

Uses:

- Managing fear.

- Control of anger.

- Gout.

- Known, chronic liver problems to support liver function in conjunction with medical treatment.

Heart #7

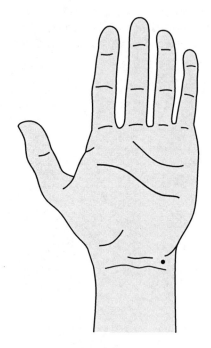

Location:

The point is on the most prominent crease of the inside of both wrists in line with the little finger. It is just below the bone that can be felt where the hand meets the wrist. Press with the tip of the thumb for 15 seconds.

Uses:

- Bad temper.
- Constipation.

Small Intestine #19

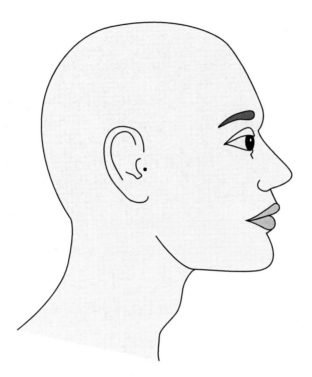

Location:

On the temporal mandibular joint which is the 'hinge' joint of the lower jaw just in front of the fleshy part of the ear that protects the ear canal itself. Press with the fingertip both sides of the head for 10 to 15 seconds.

Uses:

- Tinnitus (ringing or noises in the ears).
- Feeling of pressure in the ears.

Special Eye Points

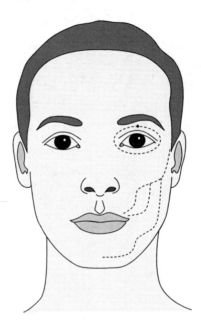

Location:

On the underside (inner edge) of the upper part of the eye socket. Before attempting to find this point make sure that your hands are clean and that your finger and thumbnails are short and smooth. With the fingertips resting on the forehead above the eye, place the tip of the thumb very gently on the inside upper edge of the bone around the eye (eye socket). You will feel a 'notch' in the bone almost above the centre of the eye. Press gently upwards with the thumb at this point. Hold the pressure for 10 seconds. May be repeated if necessary after 20 minutes.

Uses:

- Airborne allergies (hay fever, allergic rhinitis).
- Sinus problems.
- Hay fever-related eye irritation.

Summing Up

- Become aware of the difference between an acute problem and a chronic condition. Both can be treated by acupressure, though the approach may vary.

- The pressure points illustrated have an immensely long history of use.

- Never use acupressure where the skin is broken, swollen or bruised, or on an injury or the site of recent surgery.

- Learn where not to apply pressure on the body.

- When in doubt use common sense or consult a qualified practitioner.

- Familiarise yourself with the points. Summing Up

Chapter Eight

Acupressure for Animals

Using acupressure for animals

Background

It is likely that acupressure has been used for animals for as long as it has been used for people. In older societies, before mechanisation and industrialisation when the way of life was predominantly agricultural and hunter/ gatherer based, animals were very highly valued. Animals were essential for transporting goods and people, for ploughing and other work, and of course to provide food, clothing and bedding. It would have been necessary for our ancestors to use any means at their disposal to look after their livestock.

There are records in ancient China going back to around 3000 BC which mention the practice of acupuncture on the horses of the army. Engravings of cows and horses with acupuncture points marked on them have been dated to 221 BC.

'It is likely that acupressure has been used for animals for as long as it has been used for people.'

Theory

One of the basic principles of acupressure is that ki (qi) is a universal energy which flows through all things. In animals, as in humans, ki flows throughout the whole body, mostly through meridians. These are very similar to the meridians in a human being, as are the pressure points. Obviously the anatomy of animals means that there are some differences, tails for instance. The charts for animals will tend to have more variation from one source to another than human charts as well. This means that an even greater amount of intuition and sensitivity is needed with animals than with humans when finding acupressure points.

Legal matters

Before using a complementary therapy of any kind on an animal, or asking a therapist to help your animal, it is important to find out what the legal situation is in your country or state.

At the time of writing, the law in the UK with regard to using complementary therapies with animals is under review. Find out what the current law is before you proceed. A summary of the law as it stands is that owners are allowed to give whatever treatment they want to an animal as long as it does not involve intrusion into the body of the animal. You cannot even give an injection to your animal unless instructed to do so by a vet. You cannot give acupuncture to an animal unless you are a vet and are also a qualified acupuncturist.

The only therapists allowed to work on animals are physical therapists such as those practising chiropractic, physiotherapy, osteopathy, massage and acupressure. The law states that a vet must give permission for any therapy given to an animal. That means that your vet can refer you to a therapist they know and approve of.

There is nothing to stop you as the owner from learning acupressure, shiatsu or massage and applying it to your own pets.

'An even greater amount of intuition and sensitivity is needed with animals than with humans when finding acupressure points'

When is acupressure for animals useful?

As with humans, acupressure is not a substitute for professional help when an animal is injured or sick. Always seek veterinary help or advice when something is wrong with an animal that you do not understand, except for the most obvious and minor situation when you may administer emergency first aid. If a problem persists, gets worse or more complex call the vet.

Owners may find acupressure useful to relieve stress, pain and some other symptoms in their animals. This should be used only in circumstances where the underlying problems are known. Otherwise acupressure could be used, for instance, to relieve pain or to calm an animal until you can get to the vet.

Professional acupressure practitioners can help with all sorts of problems, physical, emotional and behavioural. Various kinds of acupressure are very popular for horses and dogs in the UK. Shiatsu in particular is quite widely accepted. Many courses in animal acupressure are available both for owners and professionals. Acupressure can have a role in improving the performance of show and sporting animals as well as for health problems and injuries. Remember that in the UK if you want a therapist to treat your animal you will need a referral from a vet. Elsewhere in the world please check the local law.

EFT and similar therapies work well on animals and can particularly help a distressed animal or deal with a phobia, obsessive behaviour, bad habits, etc.

Useful pressure points for dogs and horses

Basic characteristics of dogs and horses

Dogs and horses were chosen as example species for several reasons:

1. They are among the most common domesticated animals.

2. They have a long history of working with humans.

3. There are some fundamental differences between the two species:

- Horses are prey animals, dogs are hunters.

- Horses are vegetarian, dogs are omnivores but mostly carnivorous.

- Dogs have a gall bladder, horses do not – both have a Gall Bladder meridian.

- Dogs have developed a co-operative social structure for hunting in packs, horses have a different herd mentality.

4. Dogs and horses are commonly treated with acupressure.

It is useful to have these differences in mind when treating dogs or horses particularly when dealing with behavioural problems. The way that horses react in a given situation is very different from a dog because of fundamental differences in their nature.

'EFT and similar therapies work well on animals and can particularly help a distressed animal or deal with a phobia, obsessive behaviour, bad habits, etc.'

Why the pressure points were chosen

The reasons for choosing the pressure points that are described in this chapter are mostly practical ones.

The points must:

- Be useful for common problems.
- Be easy to locate.
- Have no contraindications.

The points and their uses

Dog and horse charts

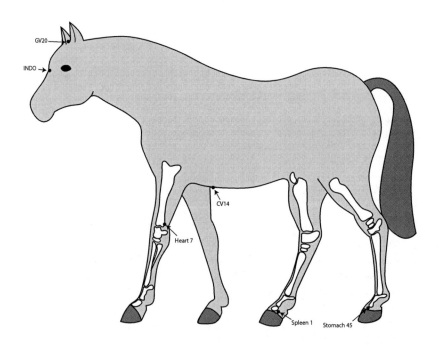

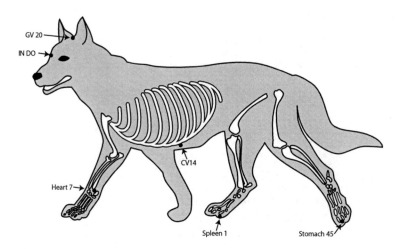

Comparison of the two charts illustrates very well how the location of points differs between two species. The points on the head and body are quite similar but the leg points differ quite a bit because of the differences between horse and dog bone structure.

The points shown on these charts are useful for calming and balancing in general as well as other specific uses. They are particularly handy for first aid when your animal is distressed or frightened.

The points

Governing Vessel #20

Location:

On the central line of the head between the ears. Press for around 10 seconds. Governing Vessel #20 is the meeting place of the Governing Vessel, Bladder, Gall Bladder, Triple Heater and Liver meridians. It is called 'Hundred Convergences' and is a very important and useful point for balancing yang energy. Simply placing the flat of the hand between the animal's ears and resting it there for a minute or so or gently patting that area can have a very calming effect.

Uses:

- Calming and balancing – any extreme behaviour, anger, fear, etc.

- Eye soreness or pain.

- May help colic and its associated pain.

In Do

Location:

On the central line of the front of the head between the eyes, one thumb's width above a line drawn between the centre of the eyes. Press with a fingertip for 10 to 15 seconds or rest the palm of your hand in this area.

Uses:

- Calming and balancing.

- Blocked nostrils or discharge.

- Sinus problems.

Heart #7

Location:

On the outside of both front legs at the level of the joint between the carpal bones and the ulnar (equivalent to the wrist on human). Press for 15 seconds both sides.

Uses:

- Calming, balancing, useful if the animal is anxious or appears to be unhappy.

- Insomnia.

- Constipation.

- Bad temper, aggressive behaviour.

Central Vessel #14

Location:

On the central line of the underside of the body. Measure halfway between the navel and the bottom point of the breastbone (xyphoid process), then measure halfway between this point and the xyphoid process again. This is CV #14. Press for 10 to 15 seconds with the fingertip. Resting the palm of the hand on this area will also help to calm the animal.

Uses:

- Control of fear, calming.
- Bronchitis, pleurisy.
- Irrational behaviour.
- Hiccups.

Spleen #1

Location dog:

Base of the claw on the innermost digit on the inside of the rear leg (both sides). Press the point for 10 seconds with the tip of the index finger. Alternatively pinch the base of the claw with the thumb and fingertips. Press on both legs.

Location horse:

Just above the top edge of the hoof, on the inside of the rear legs towards the rear of the hoof. Press both legs with the finger or thumb tip for 20 seconds.

Uses:

- Calming, especially if the animal is distressed by illness or infection.
- To boost the immune system.
- Bloated abdomen.
- Manic behaviour.

Stomach #45

Location dog:

On the inside edge of the base of the second claw from the inner rear paw (both legs). Press with fingertip for 15 seconds.

Location horse:

Just above the top edge of the rear hoof at the front of the hoof. Press with your thumb or fingertip for 20 seconds.

Uses:

- Fear.
- Mania/Depression, mood swings.
- Agitation.

EFT for animals

Principles

The basic concepts of EFT were introduced in chapter 3. One of the applications of EFT is in the treatment of animals, particularly to help with behavioural aspects. As with humans, it has been found that EFT is effective in a wide range of situations, whether emotional, mental or physical.

One of the theories underlying the more advanced applications of EFT is that all living beings are connected on an energetic level and that whatever you do to yourself you are doing to those who you are connected to. This is how surrogate and remote EFT techniques work. For instance, it may be difficult to tap on a series of pressure points on an animal because of its aggressive or skittish behaviour. Or you may not be confident about the location of pressure points on a particular animal. In such a case you can simply focus your attention on the animal, or place a hand on it to make a connection and tap the

'One of the theories underlying the more advanced applications of EFT is that all living beings are connected on an energetic level and that whatever you do to yourself you are doing to those who you are connected to.'

relevant pressure points on your own face or body. This may sound strange or far-fetched but I have personal experience of treating horses, dogs and cats with EFT in this way very effectively.

Using EFT for animals

There are many applications for EFT with animals and many different ways of applying it. The most obvious use is probably to help with emotional problems. It has also been used successfully to promote wound healing, to enhance recovery from an operation or illness, or to encourage a herd of cows to mate with a bull!

Example 1

The subject is a 3-year-old male Bichon Frisé called 'K'.

'K' is an intelligent and sensitive dog with a laid-back, friendly and happy kind of personality. One day, while in the garden, a hot air balloon came overhead and began firing its gas burner, making a loud roaring noise. 'K' became almost instantly terrified. It was obvious that he could not understand this strange object hanging in the sky, making a roaring sound like a dragon.

He ran off towards the house and wouldn't be consoled. In fact he was shaking like a leaf and crying. I began tapping on the points under his eyes (particularly good for fear) and repeating an affirmation to him, 'Even though the balloon was very scary, and I was terrified, I fully accept myself,' followed by, 'I am releasing this fear.' It became apparent that he found the tapping irritating, so I simply held the pressure points until he became a little calmer. Next I tapped some pressure points on my own fingers, while repeating the phrases in my head and focusing my attention fully on 'K'.

For a few days following his big fright, when outside, 'K' would often look up at the sky checking that no strange things were about to invade his space! Immediately after the event, even seing the moon would upset him. It took a few sessions with some reinforcing of the EFT and he got over the phobia fairly rapidly.

Example 2

The subject is a 12-year-old Gelding, Welsh Cob cross.

This horse was normally a happy, lively creature and generally well-behaved. He was treated by the vet for leg problems which had affected his ability to walk and run. The treatment was successful but the horse was still not running. At this point I was asked to treat the horse because there was no apparent physical reason why he could not run.

The horse moved quite well when led yet seemed reticently tense. It seemed to me that although he was physically better, the horse was anticipating a problem when he tried to walk or trot. In other words, he was worried that it would hurt and this was holding him back. This is not an uncommon problem in humans and animals when recovering from an injury.

I started by patting him on the GV 20 point between his ears for about 20 seconds to calm and balance his energies and to get him used to my touch. Then while repeating the phrases: 'Even though I am frightened to run, in case it hurts me, I fully accept myself' and, 'It's ok to run, it won't hurt me' I started tapping the points under the eye, at the side of the eyebrow and the collarbone points. Throughout the treatment I made sure not to look into his face or eyes and to stand to the side of the horse. This is important because horses are a prey animal and would be intimidated and scared by any confrontational body language. That would make the EFT treatment ineffective.

The owner then walked the horse down a track to see if he would trot. He did trot but seemed to still be holding back. So I repeated the tapping of the pressure points. This time I repeated the phrases: 'Pain-free running', 'Happy running', 'Fearless running'. I asked the owner to take him down the track again to see how he moved. This time the horse shot forward, the owner dropped the lead rein and he ran happily down the track, neighing as he went! He only stopped when he reached the closed gate at the end of the track and turned around to run back. The result was one happy horse and one satisfied owner.

The universal connection

In EFT, whether it is with humans or animals, it is possible to get results by speaking the affirmative phrases out loud or by saying them in your head. Some people may find this idea strange and wonder how it works. How do animals understand what you are saying? Or how do people know what you are saying inside your head? The answer is that we are dealing with a universal energy, common to all living things. When the practitioner says a phrase in conjunction with working on pressure points it sets up a pattern in his or her energy field. This creates a sympathetic pattern in the energy field of the subject which has the desired remedial effect. If that sounds too weird, just suspend your disbelief and try it, or observe it being done.

Summing Up

- Acupuncture is known to have at least a 5,000-year history of being used with animals. Acupressure would parallel this.

- Ki flows through animals just as it does through humans.

- Aquaint yourself with the various laws surrounding the treatment of animals.

- Acupressure lends itself well to easing emotional and behavioural problems in animals, EFT being particularly effective.

- Acupressure and EFT have also proven most useful in accelerating recovery from illness or injury.

Chapter Nine

Daily Routines
for Wellbeing

Approaches to health

Western strategies

In Western allopathic medicine ('conventional' medicine based on chemical medicines and surgical interventions) the emphasis has mostly been on finding cures for diseases. This is sometimes called the 'Silver Bullet' approach. The idea being that there is a specific drug or treatment which will work fully for each illness or problem. In holistic/naturopathic therapies, the need for a cure when a disease has taken hold is recognised. However, much more emphasis is placed on prevention of disease by supporting body systems and encouraging optimum health.

Good nutrition with a natural balanced diet, exercise to your level of ability, relaxation and fun, and a positive mental attitude are all part of a good preventative regime. To be fair, allopathic medicine is beginning to realise that this approach would save a lot of work and money later on.

Traditional Eastern strategies

I say 'traditional' because Western allopathic medicine has been adopted by many Eastern countries.

Traditionally, the Eastern approach to a healthy life involves:

'Good nutrition with a natural balanced diet, exercise to your level of ability, relaxation and fun, and a positive mental attitude are all a part of a good preventative regime.'

- A balanced diet. This varies with cultures and belief systems.

- Healthy exercise and lifestyle.

- Maintaining a healthy balance of the energetic systems of the body. For example, this would include tai chi, yoga, chi gong, regular massage, acupressure, shiatsu or acupuncture treatment.

- Spiritual practice like meditation or other traditional disciplines.

The role of acupressure

Acupressure has a dual role in health care, both as a treatment for symptoms and as a preventative strategy to maintain health and wellbeing. We have looked at treatment in chapter 7 using pressure points to treat symptoms and alleviate pain. Now let's look at acupressure as part of a health-promoting lifestyle.

Your daily routines

When and where

To get the most benefit from these daily routines give yourself a little time each day when you can be alone, in a quiet warm space. Perhaps you can set aside 15-30 minutes at the beginning or end of your day, or during the day when you have the house to yourself. You may wish to play some quiet relaxing music, light some incense or do whatever you need to encourage a relaxed atmosphere. Wear some loose, warm clothing, preferably in one of your favourite colours.

Before you start

Avoid doing the stretching routines i.e. 3 and 4 if:

- You have eaten within half an hour.

- You have drunk alcohol, strong tea or coffee or taken strong medication or drugs.

- You are very angry or upset.

'Acupressure has a dual role in health care, both as a treatment for symptoms and as a preventative strategy to maintain health and wellbeing.'

- You are feeling very unwell and have a high temperature.

- You have any disability, physical restrictions or problems (talk to your doctor before proceeding).

- You are heavily pregnant (talk to your doctor, midwife or other medical advisor before proceeding).

- You have a serious medical condition, heart problem, hypertension, etc. (Seek medical advice before proceeding).

If you are thirsty drink a little pure water before starting.

Waking up the ki

Often our bodies, our circulation, our breathing and our ki become stagnant. If you sit for a long while during the day or have been lying in bed for many hours the breathing becomes shallow, circulation slows and ki becomes lethargic. The same thing happens when driving a car for a long while, sitting on a train or bus or in many other sedentary situations.

So, we will begin by waking things up and gently getting the energies moving.

1. Vigorously rub the palms of your hands together and clap them a few times. Then rub them together again. Do this for a minute or so until they are starting to tingle. Now simply place your hands over your closed eyes so that the palms of the hands are cupping your eyes and the fingers are pointing upwards and resting on the forehead. This is excellent for waking up and energising the eyes or refreshing tired eyes.

   Next, stand with bare feet on a mat or rug. If it is a warm day stand outside on grass if possible. Keep your feet about the same distance apart as your hips so that there is no feeling of tension in the way you stand.

2. Let your arms hang loosely with the palms of the hands inwards, facing your thighs. Just stand like this quietly and become aware of your breathing. Gently begin to deepen the breathing by slightly increasing the length of the out breath. Breathing is through the nose, not the mouth. This filters the air as you inhale and is kinder to the lungs. As you extend the out breath the in breath will automatically become deeper to match it. Allow your breathing to gradually deepen, over the course of 20 or so *slow, even* breaths. When

'If you sit for a long while during the day or have been lying in bed for many hours the breathing becomes shallow, circulation slows and ki becomes lethargic.'

you have reached the point when you are breathing in and out fully, allow your breathing to return to normal. Do not strain or force your breathing or hold your breath. If you feel dizzy or headachey you are probably forcing the breath and trying too hard. If this happens stop and relax.

Now you can begin with some gentle stretching to warm up the muscles and improve the circulation of blood throughout the body. If you are familiar with hatha yoga or tai chi this is a good time to include a favourite exercise like 'Salute to the Sun' or a short tai chi form.

3. Otherwise, begin by slowly bringing the arms round to rest on the front of the thighs, with the palms against the thighs. Keeping the arms straight but relaxed, slowly raise them in front of the body. Continue until the arms are above the head with the palms facing forwards. While you are doing this (a few seconds) breathe in, so that when the arms reach the top you have breathed in fully. Then, breathing out slowly, lower the arms until the palms are resting on your thighs again. Throughout co-ordinate the breath with the movement. Repeat 3 times.

4. Move the palms of the hands to the side of the thighs and, keeping your arms straight but relaxed, slowly raise them out sideways from the body. Keep going until your arms are horizontal and the palms are facing downwards. Pause and breathe gently while you turn your palms to face upwards. Breathing in, raise your arms above your head until the palms meet, if possible. Breathe out, then in, maintaining the stretch. Turn the palms of the hands outwards, so the backs of the hands are together. Breathing out, lower the arms to your sides. Repeat at least twice. Do not rush.

These stretches are quite simple and gentle, and if you want to extend them or add a different range of stretches and movements then join a local yoga, tai chi or other class teaching stretching exercises that you can incorporate into your daily routine.

Respect your body

If at any time you feel any discomfort or have any difficulties while doing these exercises, stop and relax. If you have not stretched your body for a while, take your time. It is not a competition or a test. It is a way of enlivening your body, not stressing it.

Grounding and balancing your ki

In the modern world there are many distractions and a lot of sensory input constantly bombards many people. This disturbs the balance of Ki and because of the constant demands on the eyes, ears, brain and head, generally our awareness of and connection with the earth can suffer. The following routines can rectify this.

1. Depending on your ability, sit on the floor, on a cushion or a chair. Sit as upright as you comfortably can without tension building up in your back.

   Gently close your eyes and let your breathing settle. Place all the finger and thumb tips of each hand together, thus linking the hand meridians. Imagine or visualise white fibres, like roots coming out from the base of your spine. The roots travel downwards beneath you into the earth. Let them continue downward through the nourishing soil until they find a large boulder in the earth. Feel your roots wrapping themselves around the boulder and hold on to it for a few moments. Now gently unwrap the roots from the boulder and start to slowly withdraw them from the earth.

   Take your time, breath gently and eventually bring the roots back into the lower part of your spine. This is a very calming and grounding exercise and can be done in a few minutes when you are familiar with it.

   There are occasions when our energies can become scattered or it becomes hard to stay focused and grounded. You may feel overwhelmed or overloaded. This simple technique can be done in a minute or so and can bring everything down to earth and into focus.

2. Sit upright with your head erect, looking forward, shoulders relaxed (not lifted up round your ears and tense!). Reach up to take hold of your earlobes with the thumb and first finger of each hand. Keep the elbows pointing downwards. Breathe in slowly and fully and then, while breathing out, pull downwards gently but firmly on the earlobes. When you have breathed out fully stop pulling down on the earlobes and breathe in. Continue to pull down on the earlobes with each out breath. Repeat for 5 or more cycles of breathing or until calmness and a sense of stability are restored.

'There are occasions when our energies can become scattered or it becomes hard to stay focused and grounded. You may feel overwhelmed or overloaded.'

Pressure points for yin/yang balancing

This simple technique is a way of helping to restore the overall balance of yin and yang energies. It is often used as a daily self-help routine, but could easily be used on friends, partners, children or pets. I even know of one man who uses it on his sheep if they look 'under the weather'!

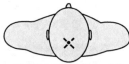
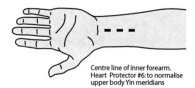

Top of the head, Governing Vessel #20: to normalise all Yang meridians

Centre line of inner forearm. Heart Protector #6: to normalise upper body Yin meridians

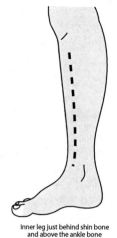

Inner leg just behind shin bone and above the ankle bone

Top of the head, Governing Vessel #20: to normalise all yang meridians.

Centre line of inner forearm, Heart Protector #6: to normalise upper body yin meridians.

Inner leg just behind shin bone and above the ankle bone, Spleen #6: to normalise lower body yin meridians.

This can be used as part of your daily routine or at any time during the day or night to help restore equilibrium.

Technique

Start with Governing Vessel #20, the point on top of the head. Using the inside of the fingers of the hand you usually write with, tap gently in a circular pattern all around the central area at the top of the head, between the ears for 20 seconds.

Next, using the inside of the fingers of the right hand gently tap the inside of the left wrist in the area illustrated incorporating Heart Protector #6. Do this for 20 seconds and then repeat on the opposite side by tapping inside of the right wrist with the fingers of the left hand.

Finally, tap the area of Spleen #6, on the inside of the leg just behind the shin bone and above the ankle bone. Gently tap the left leg with the fingers of the right hand for 20 seconds and then tap the right leg with the fingers of the left hand for the same period.

The overall effect is balancing and relaxing yet energising. If this routine is performed every day the benefits will accumulate over a period of time.

Daily routines to encourage mental and emotional wellbeing

Underlying principles

A holistic approach to health does not treat mental, emotional or spiritual aspects separately from the physical. It recognises that all four areas of life are interdependent. The acupressure, breathing, stretching and grounding routines just described benefit the whole being.

Therapies such as EFT and TFT and their derivatives, often referred to as Energy Psychology Therapies, work on the meridians in conjunction with mental, emotional and cognitive interaction. This restores a balanced state of being and dispels negative, limiting beliefs. These limiting beliefs can include phobias, lack of confidence and all those things we tell ourselves like:

'A holistic approach to health does not treat mental, emotional or spiritual aspects separately from the physical. It recognises that all four areas of life are interdependent.'

- I'm not clever enough.
- I can't draw.
- I can't paint.
- I'm too ill.
- I'll never lose weight.
- I can't swim.
- I'm not attractive, and so on.

EFT

Emotional Freedom Technique (EFT) is often applied to specific problems or a range of connected problems. However, it is possible to apply it generally to bring about an overall improvement in a holistic way.

During many years of EFT practice, I and other practitioners have found that simple daily routines of tapping on pressure points while repeating affirmations, or in some cases just tapping the points, can have very positive effects. In the case of very specific problems it is recommended that a person consult a practitioner of EFT or download the EFT manual and use it to work on themselves. In situations where there is a less specific problem or a more vague feeling that something is lacking or could be improved in one's life, experiment the following routines: the mini EFT and the fingertip tapping.

Firstly here is a reminder of the main points used in EFT:

- EB 'EyeBrow' – This point is at the end of the eyebrow nearest the nose.
- SE 'Side of the Eye' – This point is level with the outer corner of the eye just behind the bony structure that forms the orbit of the eye (not as far back as the temple but just over the bony ridge).
- UE 'Under the Eye' – This point is on the bony ridge under the eye (in line with the pupil when looking straight ahead).
- UN 'Under the Nose' – This point is between the nose and the upper lip on the vertical midline of the face.

- Ch 'Chin' – This point is situated between the lower lip and the tip of the chin (in a hollow) also on the vertical midline of the face

- CB 'CollarBone' – At the base of the throat, at about the spot where a man would knot a tie, is a soft 'notch' at the top of the breastbone. Just about 1" to the left or right of this and 1" down is a bony protuberance where the breastbone, collarbone and first rib all come together. This is the area to work on.

- BN 'Beneath Nipple' – On a man this is about 2 fingers' width below the nipple. On a woman the point is below the nipple at the point where the breast joins the chest.

- UA 'Under Arm' – Measure the width of one hand (across the biggest knuckles) from the armpit downwards. This point is on the side of the ribcage.

- Th 'Thumb point' – This point is located at the base of the thumbnail on the side furthest from the other fingers.

- IF 'Index Finger' – This point is located at the base of the index fingernail on the side nearest the thumb.

- MF 'Middle Finger' – This point is at the base of the middle fingernail on the side nearest the index finger.

- BF 'Baby or Little Finger' – This point is to be found at the base of the little fingernail at the side nearest to the other fingers.

- KC 'Karate Chop' – This is between the top of the wrist and the base of the little finger on the fleshy area at the side of the hand.

- Gamut Point – This is between the big knuckles of the ring and little fingers and about ½ an inch towards the wrist.

- Sore Spot (used in set-up) – This is the sorest spot you can find (if there is one) in the upper chest area, between the breast and the collarbone roughly halfway between the breastbone and the armpit.

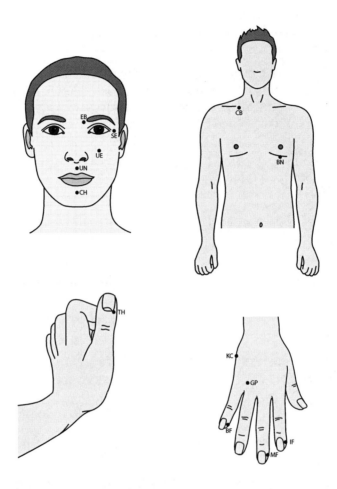

The mini EFT session

This is a simplified version of the original EFT procedure as described in Gary Craig's EFT manual. It could be added at the end of the other daily routines or could be used at any time of the day. It is probably best to perform this routine in a place and at a time when you have no distractions and are not likely to be interrupted.

The technique

First of all decide what is the most pressing problem that you would like to start working on. If you have one particular problem that is quite complex, break it down into smaller aspects.

For instance, someone may have a lack of confidence when driving a car. Doing EFT for 'fear of driving' is too vague, so it is important to break the problem down into smaller chunks. You may break it down into 'I get mixed up with the controls in my car', 'I am afraid of losing control in my car', 'I am afraid of an accident', 'I might get lost', 'I might break down', or even 'I am afraid people may think I'm an awful driver'. This technique of breaking it down can be applied to even the most complex of problems. Just start with what seems to be the biggest or the scariest aspect and work on that first.

- Firstly see if you can find a 'sore spot'. If you can then massage it with one finger or thumb for around 5 seconds. Then, referring to the pressure points in the illustration, we move into the actual treatment.

- Visualise a situation involving the aspect you want to work on. Maybe it could be something you have experienced, like losing control of your car.

- Now start tapping the points on the face. Tap each point for around 5 seconds, quite vigorously and rapidly (tap 7 times in 5 seconds). Don't tap hard enough to cause bruising though. Use your index finger for tapping all the points and you can do one side of the face or both sides, as you wish.

- Tap in the order: eyebrow, side of eye, under eye, under nose, and finally chin. Visualise the situation as before and see how you feel. If the treatment is effective you will have difficulty feeling or visualising the problem, or you may simply feel indifferent to it, with no emotional involvement. If this is the case continue tapping with the points further down the body. Start with the collarbone points, then the underarm and beneath nipple points. Tap in the same way as the face points.

- Stop and re-visualise the problem to test if it has gone. If it has you are finished, if not then move on to tapping the hand points, using the same technique. Tap in the order: thumb, index finger, middle finger, baby finger, gamut point, and finally karate chop point.

- If you get an opportunity, test in real life to see if the problem has gone away (not necessarily at that moment). If you still have a problem repeat the procedure the next day. If it has gone move on to the next aspect of your problem.

Slowly, day by day, work through any problems that may be holding you back in your life. If you feel you need it, seek out a local class to learn more about EFT or read one of the many publications or online guides that are available.

Fingertip tapping

This is a much simplified EFT technique that I have taught successfully to many people. It is very adaptable for all sorts of problems and is easily incorporated in your daily routines. If you have time for nothing else, use this, it takes less than a minute.

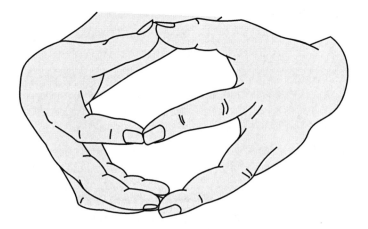

Make yourself as comfortable and relaxed as possible, take a few breaths and think about the problem or aspect of a problem that you want to work on. Start to tap your fingertips together firmly and at the rate of around two or three taps a second.

Then repeat out loud three times, slowly, a suitable positive affirmation dealing with the problem. Using the car driving example with one of my favourite affirmations might go something like: 'Even though I am afraid I might have a car accident, I fully accept myself and I am letting go of this fear' or 'I call upon my mind, body and spirit to do whatever they need to do to help me let go of this fear.' Keep working at it daily in this simple way.

If you can't think of any problems to work on (or if you have fixed them all!) then try this for simplicity. Tap your fingertips together as previously described for around 30 seconds every day while repeating the affirmation: 'Every day and in every way, I am better and better and better.'

'Every day and in every way, I am better and better and better.'

Summing Up

■ Western and Eastern approaches and attitudes to health and vitality vary.

■ Daily attention to your sense of wellbeing is recommended.

■ Breathe well and stretch your body to encourage a harmonious flow of ki energy.

■ Grounding and earthing yourself makes you feel more stable and centred.

■ Make daily routines part of your self-care.

■ Some complex problems may need breaking down into smaller aspects. Approach each one individually.

■ Take your time and keep things simple.

Help List

EFT – Emotional Freedom Technique

EFT Training

www.eft-courses.org.uk/learn-eft-manual.html
Free download of the EFT manual.
Contacts for EFT training and groups worldwide are numerous on the Internet.
Look for contacts in your locality.

World Centre for EFT

www.emofree.com
The website of the founder of EFT, Gary Craig. A new EFT manual/tutorial is to
be published in 2012 and will be available from this website.

Jin Shin Jyutsu

Jin Shin Jyutsu UK

www.jsj.org.uk
Seminars and other activities in UK.

Practitioners

Denis Jevon

Acupressure, applied kinesiology and EFT practitioner, dowser, therapeutic
masseur and writer.
Based in Shropshire, UK
Email: denis@phonecoop.coop

Tui Na

www.tuinauk.com
Practitioners and courses in the UK.

Seated Acupressure Massage

Seated Acupressure Massage and Onsite Massage (UK)

www.aosm.co.uk/
Offers comprehensive training in acupressure chair massage with a slant towards onsite massage.

Western School

Glasgow Caledonian University
6 Carrick Avenue, Ayr, Ayrshire, Scotland KA7 2SN
Tel : 01292 285609
www.westernschool.co.uk
Acupressure chair massage courses based in Scotland

Shiatsu

British School of Shiatsu

Unit 3 Thane Works
Thane Villas, London
Tel: 020 7700 3355
www.britishschoolofshiatsu.co.uk
UK-based school of shiatsu.

Ohashiatsu

www.ohashiatsu.org/us
The style of shiatsu developed by internationally famous Sensei Ohashi.

The Shiatsu Society (UK)

Shiatsu Society (UK)
PO Box 4580
Rugby
Warwickshire
CV21 9EL
Tel: 0845 130 4560
www.shiatsusociety.org
Helpful for finding practitioners or training.

Zen Shiatsu

1st Floor, 68 Great Eastern Street
London, EC2A 3JT
Tel: 070 0078 1195
www.learn-shiatsu.co.uk

TFT – Thought Field Therapy

Roger Callahan

www.rogercallahan.com
Website of Roger Callahan, founder of TFT. Lots of useful information.

TFT in the UK

www.thoughtfieldtherapy.co.uk
Website listing therapists and training in UK and Ireland

Note:

This is a small selection of contacts for seeking both training and treatments. There are many directories listing complementary therapies, including acupressure-based therapies on the Internet. Because new resources become available daily, it is a good idea to use your favourite search engine to find what is available in your country or area.

All efforts have been taken to ensure that these details are correct at the time of publication. The author has no connection with any of the contacts given.

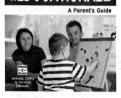
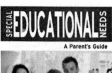
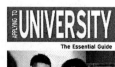
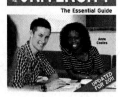
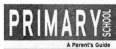
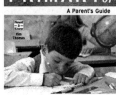
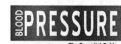
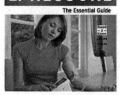
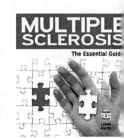